Kim

So, Thanks [illegible],

Michael J Ferguson

Carry the Message!

PLAGUE
NO MORE

Plague No More:

A Modern Odyssey of Courage and Recovery

Copyright ©2014 Michael J. Ferguson

ISBN: 978-1-940769-18-9

Publisher: Mercury HeartLink

Albuquerque, New Mexico

Printed in the United States of America

www.PlagueNoMore.com

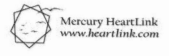

Mercury HeartLink
www.heartlink.com

PLAGUE NO MORE

A Modern Odyssey
of Courage and Recovery

Michael J. Ferguson

PLAGUE NO MORE

for Mason and Ruth,
my messenger angels

Plague
No More

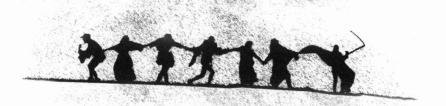

INTRODUCTION

Few people know that at least three million of us die each year from infectious diseases.

One particular killer is caused by a bacillus called *Yersinia. Pestis*. Over the course of several centuries it has taken over 250 million human lives, and is still doing so today, about a thousand a year. Unlike other diseases, there is no inoculation for it, and it is mutating to the point where conventional antibiotics may not successfully stop the next pandemic. In the United States it sometimes goes undiagnosed, most untreated patients dying of pneumonia.

In the Middle Ages its occurrence changed history, bringing about the fall of an empire, rise of a powerful theocracy, and changes in medical interventions.

Although research abounds on the history, course and treatment of this disease, there are hardly any accounts from survivors. This is one.

IT BEGINS

On August 16, 2006, I spent my 60th birthday in a hospital in Albuquerque, New Mexico dying. For ten days not even the World Class Infectious Disease Team could diagnose the cause. Strangely, I awoke that day with tubes hanging out of my arm and a whooshing sound from my nose. Squinting was all I could do, having to tilt my head side-to-side to focus on anything. God, my body felt so heavy, like I was made of concrete. When I tried to lift my right hand, it felt tied to the bed; but it wasn't. What the hell happened? That's oxygen in my nose. Why? I was breathing okay, wasn't I?

Then the glare of the lights was so bright it took every bit of strength I had to try to raise an arm to cover my eyes. I couldn't. These eyes didn't seem to want to work either. It all just didn't seem right. Plus my body ached all over. Now the room started to spin. I barely made out the shape of my brother before I dozed off again, to some weird dream I knew well when I was in it, but could barely describe it when I awoke:

There I was on a high hill in some kind of a vehicle, headed down, like on a roller coaster, holding on for dear life. At the bottom I was slowly cruising through a quaint town neighboring the one I grew up in.

A dream is like that . . . almost a recognizable reality, but not quite. Some say the unconscious is stimulated by the events of waking moments. In that room I just wanted to go home. *Ouch! Taking more blood? What am I, a pincushion?*

Nothing like this had ever happened before—no major accidents or surgeries. Well, once in high school I was hospitalized for a few days. I resolved not to go back again—and I hadn't, until now. It all seemed more like a scene on a TV medical show like *House* or *ER*, programs I would have quickly flipped through. Yet that ICU room was just like you see them: stainless steel, gauges and tubes coming out of the wall, monitor screens blipping.

Then there was that alcohol/antiseptic odor. Smells are that way for me; they register memories. I've always been a guy who would smell things. Nosey, I guess.

As I went in and out of consciousness, there was an endless procession of medical people asking me the same questions over and over: What had happened in the last few days? Who was my primary-care physician? Had I eaten any unusual foods? Been around farm animals or rodents?

My brain wasn't exactly firing on all eight cylinders, nor was I in the mood for interrogation. I shot back, "No, I can't remember doing anything different in the last week (hell, my remember-er wasn't operational, either). No, I don't have a primary-care physician. Mostly I don't like doctors." (I'm sure that went over big). "Now that rodent thing . . ." And I nodded off.

Back in that little town, again—maybe Perrysburg, Ohio—pedaling my bicycle off to the swimming pool a couple of miles down the road. Where'd that pack of dogs come from??? Gotta go faster. Now I'm in the water, gasping for air as I try to grab the side after a big guy shoved me in. He thought it was funny.

Back in the room again. They covered my mouth with a breathing mask, and for a moment I struggled. *Thank god my brother Dan is here. I'll be OK, now. Except he's looking worried. That scares me. My eyes are wet. He's wiping them dry.* That's how it's been between us. We take care of each other, though I'm ten years his senior. Last I remembered we were in the ER.

When we were growing up he was a bothersome pain-in-the-ass whose diapers I changed, the old cloth type, long before the throwaways. He became a risk taker. By the time he was six or seven he'd been knocked unconscious a few times. Once when we were kids, Mom was looking out the kitchen window at the recently constructed city high school. It was right outside of our back gate, built in the cornfield we played in. All at once, she screamed, really scaring me. Dan was standing on the gym roof, a good 40 feet off the ground. Mom was out of her mind with fear. He waved. I bolted out our back gate, sprinted across the field, shimmied up the drain pipe and grabbed him. Now it was his turn to save me.

He was the athletic one, track mostly. I learned to run foot races from him. We reconnected after he finished college when he went to work at the hometown bread company, hoping to make some quick money. He had no real plan. It didn't take much—a couple of bucks waved in his face and the promise of a cross-country road trip—to enroll him in a road trip back to Montana where I lived. We were off, as Mom would say, like a dirty shirt. No thought of hospitals back then.

Early on in that life-or-death drama, a woman showed up at my bedside. A physician with the Bernalillo County Health Department, she asked if I could pay attention for a few minutes. The interrogations commenced. What else had I been doing? Where else had I been? It was that old scientific method, but she was kind enough. The direction of the conversation led me to believe I might have gotten something serious from working in the woods. She mentioned rodents. Someplace in that nether zone between sleep and not, I got drowsy. Then the thoughts came. *Could it have been that old Airstream? Could a simple act like that change my life?*

I awakened to her light touch on my shoulder. "You just muttered something about an old trailer. Were you in one recently?"

"Yes, my friend's, just down the road from me."

"I have your address. We're going to set some traps there. I'll be back in a week to see you. You're in good hands, now."

Barely hearing her, I nodded off again.

Joe. Big silver trailer. Sunny day. Let's clean it out. Load logs. Drive to Bubba's. Nap. Hard time getting home . . .

I was in a fog and this was too much clear information. Save this for her next visit when I'm more lucid. *Sorry, doc, I gotta go.* Unconscious I went.

There was that antique 25-foot trailer. It was the central treasure on a little piece of New Mexico heaven just a stone's throw from mine.

Joe and I were in the high desert at 7,300 feet, sunshine on a beautiful summer day. Pals for 25 years, we shared a common vision of a creative high desert life. One might call him an old hippie, except that he hasn't done enough drugs, been unemployed or divorced enough times to fit the category. Sometime in the early '80s we met in a seminar offered by an educational organization whose goal was transforming lives. Friendships start that way, sharing of a common interest. In that workshop he stood up in response to a question and I liked what he said. I sought him out. We talked. The adventure commenced.

Over the years I've tried to analyze this friendship, but every organizer I used left me more confused. I like his integrity. He lives by honorable values and is an academic who treasures ideas. So do I. As an artist he draws, paints, plays music and epitomizes creativity. He is also a guy's guy who loves sports. I'm not. His insights are well thought out, not necessarily mainstream. And that sense of humor, though offbeat, causes me to laugh. We do a lot of that.. Our friendship has remained steady during the more than twenty years that he moved around—to Washington, D.C., Lubbock, Texas, and Muncie, Indiana— as he climbed the next steps up his career ladder. He's a Ph.D. professor of Architecture now. Strangely, I stayed in one place, building my own six-sided home in the mountains outside of Albuquerque. It's designed after a traditional Navajo home, a Hogan.

A couple of years before this hospital trauma, Joe and I were walking together down the fairly deserted road past my place when Joe saw a FOR SALE sign on a piece of land. Not more than a day or two later he had purchased it.

Several times a year he visits and we collaborate on materializing an idea. We also love second-hand shops. Our favorite place is Coronado Salvage in Albuquerque's South Valley. Without saying so, our goal has been to assemble odds and ends, connecting them here and there, making inventive shelters.

His first acquisition on the property he bought was a shiny, 25-foot mobile home, purchased at a "steal." Built in the '60s, it was heavy, still holding together well, and fix-up-able. Once it had arrived and been ooh-ed and ahhh-ed over, the touchup began. We did a thorough cleaning, including removing nested rodents. In retrospect, perhaps I should have dumped the drawer made into a home by the mice before reaching in and lifting them out. Rather than brutally evicting the critters, my attempt at some kind of consideration might have been costly. Though I was wearing gloves, something might have made its way up my left arm, biting me just below the shoulder. I had no sense of an intruder. Unbeknown to me, that might have set me on a life-altering trip.

I came to, flat on my back in the Intensive Care Unit.

Then I remembered: the day after I helped Joe something wasn't right. After eating a sandwich at noon I got sick and threw it up in the bushes. That was weird. It was a Friday. The next day I delivered some logs into town to a friend who intended them as posts on his porch. I felt nauseous. When I arrived at his house I went in and collapsed on his couch for a two-hour nap. He unloaded the logs and asked me if I was out late the night before, as it was unusual for me to sleep during the day. No! But on the way home I could barely keep my eyes open. After the thirty-mile drive, I literally fell out of my truck and crawled to my couch.

When I was unaccounted for on Monday at a remodel job, my buddy Kent realized how unusual it was for me to not show up or at least call in, and decided to check up on me after work. After rousing me, he said he found me unconscious on the front walkway. I had been out there for 48 hours. Thank God it was summer.

When I awoke I was groggy and asked Kent to call my brother Dan. He found the number in my phone. Dan came immediately. I said it was just a case of flu. I hobbled to his car in a bathrobe and he drove to the closest Emergency Room. I passed out in a chair, probably for hours. When I came to, they determined that I was dehydrated, gave me $150 worth of fluids, and sent me stumbling home. "If you're not better tomorrow, you're going back," Dan said.

The next day I wasn't better and we did go back. This time I got admitted.

Sometime later, probably that night, I awoke in an ICU with a young man asking me to sign an admission form. Hardly able to hold the pen, I made an X. I had no idea what had happened. Neither did any of the medical staff. It seemed I was told that a reaction to sulfur caused a complete body rash, including red eyes. I overheard a visitor say, "He looks dead." Then someone suggested that I should do a Living Will. *Uh oh! This was serious.* As I scanned around the room I saw my brother Dan, looking really scared. I'd only seen that look one other time, when we laid our motorcycles down riding in rainy weather years before, coming down a mountain. We were driving slowly, so no injuries. Upon getting up we hugged each other. He said: "Man, you barely missed my melon."

Now in the ICU, my head fell to the left. Several feet away, was a large sliding door to the corridor. Groggy as I looked through it, I saw something strange. *What is that?*

JUST BEFORE IT HAPPENED

Life had been going along steadily for a few years. My house was built in 2000; it was cozy, and I was able to make the payments on time. My fairly new career in construction was progressing. Running commercial construction projects for a company in Los Alamos, after receiving a two-year degree in Project Management in 1996, I worked hard. The compensation was good. After that, picking up small jobs here and there came easily enough. Working in construction fulfilled a part of me that had been dormant for years.

Ever since I was a kid I've loved to build things. My dad was always after me to return tools to his bench after I'd used them. He wasn't a guy who was particularly handy, nor did he have a lot of gumption for projects. But in a pinch he could fix a thing or two. He'd crafted a bench and had a few tools. I knew they were his, but since I used them more than he did, I treated them like they were mine. Actually, he'd rather have been reading mystery books and watching TV, or listening to baseball on the radio, especially the Cleveland Indians; but he always provided for our family, and was a good model of an honorable man.

We lived in Maumee, Ohio, a burgeoning suburb of Toledo, in the 1950's. Once I recall returning home from a walk by a newly constructed home site in our neighborhood, with a treasured handful of scrap wood. Using Dad's tools, I fashioned a riverboat steamer, nailing progressively smaller blocks of wood onto each other. Painted and outfitted with miniature sailors, I took it to a nearby pond. I proudly pushed it out to sea. It sank. I went home undaunted. As I aged, crafting an education replaced woodworking.

In the '70s, my wife, Jeanette, and I sold our goods in Ohio, filled a pick-up truck with necessities, and moved to Montana. Having purchased ten acres of land the year before, the following year, 1974, we camped out for a summer while building our log cabin, just like early settlers. We lived there for several years. That was real adventure for a city kid.

Some local boys were adept with mechanical things and convinced me to try my hand at wrenching. An old Volkswagen became my first victim. I studied a handbook on the subject and actually became sort of, kind of, handy with tools–at least enough to know that I wasn't meant to live with grease under my fingernails. But I did learn things I had never learned as a kid. Those "hippies" also opened the door to the darkness with that "funny looking home-rolled cigarette" (dope).

Sidetracked, I took a walk on the wild side for a few years. It initiated a way of living that ultimately cost me the love of a good woman and probably a few years off of my life. I could only live that way for a while – I knew I was headed for a fall. So I loaded my Volkswagen van with my goods and put my motorcycle in a trailer. My faithful canine traveling companion, Buck, climbed into the van with me and off we went. It was 1980, and I was on my own, headed south to New Mexico.

By 2006 I'd quit the wild side of drugs and alcohol use more than seventeen years earlier. I had solid friendships and was attempting to live honorably. Around me there were a few fellows living useful lives and trying to stop their craziness, as well. In fact, Kent, who found me passed out that fateful day, had been for a couple of months off of the "sauce." His gesture of concern saved my life. I had actually done the same for him two months earlier when I scraped him off of the curb, helped him "dry out," and put him to work with me.

Since "cleaning up," over the years I'd found my way to a spiritual life, praying daily for others, finding strength to keep doing right things. It had gotten easier. In fact, there were many moments and extended periods when I was at peace.

At first when that happened I found myself uneasy with the calm. For as long as I could remember I had been restless, irritable, discontented and worried. Terror, frustration, bewilderment, and despair were my constant companions, even as I tried my best to stay one step ahead. Though I had been raised in a good Irish Catholic family, future alcohol abuse was planted in my genes. Both of my grandfathers had died drunks. Uncles and cousins were afflicted, and aunts had married alcoholics. Growing up the oldest of seven, I tried to watch over them, yet make my own way. I had put myself through college in the late '60s, then got a graduate degree in Behavioral Sciences with appropriate licenses to help others. Somehow I couldn't quite help myself, though. Tension and stress kept running my life. Prior to age 42, relaxing without external assistance had hardly ever happened.

Finally, on April 15, 1989 enough was enough, and I put the "plug in the jug." Stopping alcohol and any remnants of illegal drug use was a rebirth.

So, with my 60th birthday approaching in August 2006, a week earlier five younger siblings had come from back east to join my brother Dan from Albuquerque and me. A grand party was enjoyed by all. Although they were really coming for brother Dan's wedding, I delighted in the fact that this was the first time all seven of us had been together in New Mexico, 25 years after I'd left Ohio. The same week they arrived, my mom's brother, Jim, came to visit from Seattle. We all played tourist, ate good food and laughed a lot. This was the week before I was in the hospital dying of God-knew-what.

MORE HOSPITAL ADVENTURES

As I nodded in and out of this world I noticed things. My mentor, Keith, seemed to be present right from the first day. At a time ten years earlier he had been in the right place at the right time when I needed him. His welcoming warmth, good ear and wise counsel over the years helped me through numerous self-induced debacles. A few years older than I, he has filled a special space in my life. Neither his strong religious preference nor politics fit mine, but these differences are minor compared to what we bring into each other's lives.

He's been the older brother I never had, real family to me. Being an oldest child, I had no older sibling to "show me the ropes" of life. He's done that on so many occasions. A 6-foot-plus man with long arms for hugs, a booming voice for a loud, deep laugh, and penetrating blue eyes for a soft "I love you," I treasure him. His comfort helped save my life.

Early on it was clear to me that Keith was around to assist me, but later I was able to help him. When he and his sister had a major falling-out over health care for their ailing mother, he was livid. Actually, it was more like a rage preceding murder, and I was able to see him through that with no homicide, nor even an assault charge.

Aside from Keith, there were the medically dressed bodies who regularly scurried about, taking blood and vital signs. Some were kind, some were not. Through my fog I remember a nurse showing up with a horse needle and an attitude. I said, "You're not going to use that on me, are you?"

"I sure am, now close your eyes. This won't hurt much." It did.

Soon after, I awoke with a group of doctors clustered around the foot of the bed. It must have been the second or third day. *What do they want?* All I could do was lie there in that pathetic condition having a silent conversation with myself–it was too much trouble to talk. They did their undertone doctor-speak, one hand rubbing their chins, the other hand supporting the first at the elbow. To me it looked like a gaggle of geese with ducklings tagging along. They didn't seem to know what was wrong, either. I could barely interpret the "doctorese." One said, "When you have an issue, get more tissue." *Real cute,* I mused back at them silently.

On Tuesday, I was 60, as a nurse in that room inserted a tube into my pee-er because I couldn't even get out of bed. *That really, really hurt. Happy Birthday, Michael!* Usually one gets a cake.

Someone wanted me to sign a paper, again, so they could stick something in my right forearm. I struggled to write another X. More fluids needed to be pumped into me at the same time. I hesitated to approve. My brother explained that it was necessary, so I let them do it.

The phone rang. Family calling. Under the influence of medication, I was later told that I was yelling loudly—it was, after all, long distance. My baby sister, Mary, who works at Ohio State University in the veterinary medicine area, was on the line. She's really bright and I gave permission for the doctors to talk to her. That's when I found out they really didn't know what I had, or what had me. Even so, it sure was good to hear Mary's voice. We've always been close. She invented brutal honesty and can tell crude jokes like a Marine, but there is a soft side to her, too. We laugh a lot. It doesn't take much for her to see something humorous in almost any situation; and point it out. After I told her how much weight I was losing since I couldn't eat, she commented that this was a great diet plan. Right.

Lots of friends visited. Apparently word had gotten around that I wouldn't be alive long. Keith told me later that he thought they came to say goodbye.

Once when I was finally alone, I suddenly realized how scared I was. There were frequent moments when tears would run down my cheeks. Memories of good buddies' faces floated in and out, as did I.

During a quiet period when I was awake, there was a short, brown-skinned lady mopping and cleaning up. That dark figure outside the sliding glass door was still there. I asked her who that was. Above her facemask, her dark eyes looked intently at me. She came close, took my hand in hers, bent to my ear and I heard, "God, please help this man." I drifted off.

Dino's Gift

During my first week in the hospital, most of my daily energy was spent in breathing, sporadic eating, turning over in bed, and switching channels on the TV. One morning after mandatory medical visits from doctors, nurses (to check my vital signs), and phlebotomists, I heard a familiar greeting, "Howdy, partner." Only one person announces himself that way, Dino Mike. He was dubbed "Dino" because of his affinity for studying science and geology and for excavating the fossils of extinct creatures. We had met nine years earlier upon my return from Saudi Arabia. Being a bit stocky, his jaunty movements reminded me of a bodyguard or Samurai. There was nothing slow about him at all. He was always engaged in some interesting endeavor like paleontology, chemistry, or astronomy, and dedicated to the lives of his grown children and grandchildren. Politics riled him, so he volunteered for various election campaigns. On top of this he is an accomplished musician, teaching band (lots of instruments) to elementary school kids. Something one of my first mentors said to me applied to him, "You've just got too damned many interests". Years before a therapist had diagnosed him with Adult Attention Deficit Disorder. His assessment was that he had an "intense interest in a lot of things." Too much of that can make a person nuts, I know from experience. Like many other recovering people, he had been on and off medication. We were roughly the same age, and both making an effort toward an honorable life. Being cohorts in the ongoing struggle to balance care for ourselves with care for other, we seemed to show up in each other's lives just when one of us needed assistance. I did not know the gift he was bearing this visit.

Personal grooming was low on my list of priorities, surviving being the highest that first week. When Dino came close to my bed we shook hands, smiled, then he rubbed the back of his hand across my face and said, "You're looking a little scraggly, man. Care for a shave?" That was close to the last thing on my mind.

"Sure, I guess. But you'll have to get a razor and stuff from the nurses' station."

"Let me see what I can find," he muttered as he turned on his way out of the door.

I started to reflect, then. I was one who had done so much for others, mostly because I wanted to. There had been times when others asked something of me and I didn't provide it. I was a generous giver when I wanted to be, so who was it really for? Now people were doing for me. I had never received a shave from another person, even a barber. This was going to be different, all right. Shaving is a real personal thing. Women talk about things like that, guys don't. Hair on the face is a rite-of-passage for a young man.

My first razor, in the 60's, was a hand-me-down electric one from my dad. Electric appliances seem to make things easier. Besides, I didn't know how to lather my face nor drag a razor across it. I know why guys grow a beard! It is work to scrape stubbles off of tender skin. That was then. Before I could nod off for a nap, Dino returned, disposable razor in hand, proudly holding up an institutional mini-sized shaving cream can. The party was on. Needless to say both of us were extra careful, no cuts and a clean face being the result. Once again I was touched at the act of kindness. He was just one of so many who took time from busy schedules to drive to the hospital, wrangle for a parking spot, follow the clues to my room and visit. One day ten people performed that act of generosity. Amazing.

———

THOSE I TRUSTED

Did you ever awaken and not know where you were, or what was real? Sometimes I just couldn't tell. Drugs and fever did that. One measure I used was the kindly medical people who cared for me: I knew they were real. They just seemed like angels to me. Most days I was so low on energy that I could only smile and say thank you.

Right from the first day, Randy the RN who seemed to be in charge, was there. His soft-spoken ways and professionalism gave me confidence. In his left hand there was that palm-sized black unit where he entered responses to questions. I was sure my medical life and the answer to what was wrong with me were in there. I strained like a little kid to see what was in it. Once I asked him what was wrong with me. He touched my hand softly, locked eyes with mine, and replied, "We don't really know, Michael, but you're medically stable and I'm here with you. You're OK now."

His personable approach and his willingness to tell me the truth helped me a lot. I relaxed and believed what he said. A deep trust was planted at that moment. Every time we spoke it was reinforced. The room became softer when Randy entered, and I didn't feel so alone against my illness when he was there.

The same was true for Dr. Red. His casual jetting in and out was almost unnoticeable. At some point he must have talked to one of the score of people coming to visit me. During a lull he returned to ask me about my previous drug and alcohol abuse, and he sounded sincerely interested in me and my situation. I was touched to tears, again. As I found out later, he was knowledgeable in this area, having treated many alcoholics. He understood.

Both Randy and Dr. Red had heard my delirious chatter. Once I was asked if I knew where I was. I told them I was in Toledo Hospital (where I had once been as a teenager). So one day I took a chance and asked them about the elusive shadow in the corridor. I remember Randy's quick sideward glance at the door when I asked him. What he said next did surprise me: "When do you see it?"

"A couple of times a day," I said. "It's not like a person, more like a dark moving blur when I catch sight of it."

"I haven't run into it," Randy replied, "but I have to tell you that others have mentioned this to me. I'll have Security check it out." Then he said quietly, "You are safe." I believed him, and I stopped worrying for the moment. But a couple of times when I was shuttled around in a wheelchair for tests, I thought I saw something out of the corner of my eye, over there when we turned right, or going to get yet another x-ray of my chest. Again in the MRI trailer, out back, I could have sworn something was present. I kept wondering what it was. On a one-to-ten scale of concern it was only about a three.

Other issues were more important, like trying to walk. About the second day a couple of hospital staff tried to get me out of bed to test my legs. They coaxed me up, placed a walker in front of me, gently prodding me to take a step. I couldn't move. That's when the thought came: *I'll never walk, again.* I had no energy; I could barely hold myself upright. Every muscle and bone in my body hurt when I moved. Even flus and colds were never like this. As I leaned on the metal bracing to try to take a step I heard myself say, "Oh, shit!" The aide exhaled quickly, trying to hold back a chuckle, which he knew was inappropriate.

What really troubled me was the experience of lifelessness. I had never felt so weak. Mostly, I have always had an abundance of energy; I had get-up-and-go all the time. An old girlfriend once said that she would never be bored hanging around me. If I wasn't doing something, I was scheming to. Now I could hardly move. It made sense to me later, when an MRI person explained that she had never seen anyone with infection such as mine everywhere in the body.

Only one other time had I experienced this sort of helplessness. That was forty-five years earlier when I was in a hospital as a teenager having some kind of cyst removed. Since then, a good long run of health had made me forget how it felt to be helpless. Now, to move my head or roll over in bed took all the strength I had. What happened to the guy I had been a week earlier, who could work ten hours a day doing hammer, saw and nail? Gone. "I guess it's all over," I muttered to myself in despair.

COULD THIS HAVE BEEN WHAT HAPPENED?

When Bubba asked if there were trees on my land that he could use to make posts for his porch, I said, "Sure." We'd been friends for a couple of years and shared the same first name, but he preferred to be called Bubba. We met through a non-drinking group and our spiritual connection was strong; we were more like brothers who liked each other.

A couple of decades earlier he'd lived on the streets of Washington, D.C. That was a few years after he mustered out of the infantry from Vietnam, hit the skids, got divorced, and found heroin. He was thin and wiry, and I couldn't imagine this smiling wise-cracker as a down-and-out street junkie. But when we shared some of our experiences, strength seemed to come to us. Together we found that we could deal with life's difficulties with hope. Rarely do you meet someone who feels almost immediately like family, but that's what Bubba is. We'd both been construction supervisors, each loved our own solitude, and were deep down loners—he a lot more so than I. Throw in mutual divorce histories, admiration for women, enjoyment of a hard day's work, and you have the makings of a good friendship.

There were times, though, when Bubba went over the top with rage. A series of seemingly insignificant events could put him in a place of out-of-control anger. He would rail on and on for hours at a time about bad drivers or arrogant politicians. This was a monthly occurrence. Once when we were taking a break on a job site in town, I asked him if he went to the Veterans Hospital for medical care. He said, "Of course."

When I suggested that he might want to get PTSD screening at his next appointment, he got very upset. This diagnosis was something I knew about. In earlier years I'd been a social worker and had had some dealings with veterans suffering from Post Traumatic Stress Disorder. Since the end of the Vietnam War, more men have died at home from suicide than were killed on foreign soil. I was worried about him and about his resistance to seeking treatment.

"Why, do you think I have some problems?" He sounded angry at me for having asked the question. Because he'd never been arrested since he'd sobered up, had raised two healthy sons, had a successful career, and was now a realtor with his own investment property, there appeared no evidence of dysfunction. (Years later, when he did finally have a screening the interviewing psychologist canceled several hours of other appointments to spend time with him. Bubba told me that he had never felt so understood before.)

One of our conversations had been about God and death. Two years before we met, he had discovered he was diabetic— the hard way. He went into a coma and was hospitalized. While unconscious he had died and "gone into the Light." Upon being revived, he was disappointed to be back in his body. He told me that as a result of that near-death experience, he is just biding his time, waiting to go back to that place he had experienced briefly. This desire we also shared, for I have never, at my core, wanted to be here. Ever since I learned about Spirit, as a kid, I wanted more of that, and to be "there." And what I was looking for seemed not to be that available in this world, where we have to live with other human beings. It appeared to me that humans in general are really not that trustworthy, nor profoundly loving of each other. To escape the "here" with all its shortcomings, I turned to alcohol and drugs. Those substances temporarily put me "there," but sooner or later I had to come back here. (A mentor once told me, "They call alcohol 'spirits' for a reason, Michael.") Bubba and I agreed that we are spirits having a human experience, longing to go home– wherever, whatever that is.

So, ending up at Bubba's house with a load of logs when I was incubating my illness was no surprise. What followed shouldn't have been, either. Daily during my hospitalization I would awaken at some point to find him at my bedside. He'd always say, "Hey, buddy, we're still here, huh?" I'd always smile and sometimes shed a tear. He gave me encouragement to keep living; but at some level I really didn't want to. Little did I know that I would come to a dramatic choice about this as I faced my dark night of the Soul.

In the early morning hours that second day I was jolted awake. Tears were in my eyes over a vividly remembered dream. I was in a dark corner with some sense of a portal beckoning me. Clearly, to this day I recall saying, "I don't wanna go!" That was a life-altering decision. In our lives there are a few clear markers: graduations, marriages, first jobs, etc. That one was for me.

With that declaration I embarked on a new level of being here in this life. The next morning I asked my brother to bring me a copy of the Serenity Prayer. As chance would have it someone had just given him a Celtic cross with that prayer inscribed on it. He brought it to me, and I clutched it often. That "dream" interrupted my almost life-long depression. Sometimes it happens that way.

As a kid I dealt with disappointments by hiding under a bed wrapped in a blanket. We all have to find a way to cope with discouragements; mine was to escape.

For sure, life hadn't met my expectations. It became most clear when I was facing an uncertain future upon graduation from college in January 1968. The Vietnam War was escalating. College pals were dying. I was really scared. I remember a buddy calculating the amount of munitions per square foot in Vietnam. My dad, a World War II veteran, only shook his head, saying "War is hell" and "I'd never go again," though he never told me what to do. Strangely, I was plucked from that hell, another story of being watched over. The Creative Intelligence destined me to not have to experience war, this lifetime.

Shortly thereafter I found reasons to live: my marriage to Jeanette at age 24, followed by graduate school, and then by a move to Montana. Living in a tent for a summer and building our own log cabin were happy-making distractions. Depression was assuaged until I started experimenting with drugs and alcohol. That precipitated a divorce at 31 and a reopening of the question: "What am I doing here?" Jeanette was right to leave. I was crazy. It still broke my heart; divorce always does it to somebody.

From that time on, I was running frantically, trying to find a reason to live. That is what substance abuse does: anesthetizes the pain of living and makes the user feel better. Mostly, I would always return to sadness and depression. For another twelve years I experienced mounting discouragement, and kept chasing adventures to keep going. When I could no longer stay ahead of my own frantic pace, I stopped fueling it. Once that happened I came face-to-face with myself: unmet expectations, no satisfying connection to the Creative Spirit of the Universe, shame, guilt, frustration, and despair. It's hell to have to grow up at age 42. But we all have to do it sometime.

Still, for years I regularly thought about stepping into the street in front of a semi or putting a gun in my mouth or veering just a hair at 100 mph on my motorcycle into a bridge abutment; or taking myself out on pills. I truly understand how this happens to us. In a saner moment I promised myself that I'd call all of my siblings to say goodbye before I attempted suicide. Once, on a very, very deep-pit night, I started to call them. I'd have to make six phone calls before the act. I began with my brother, Dan, to whom I'd grown most close, and who lives in the same city as I. After a few words we both started crying, then he made me promise to get help. I promised. But I didn't get help. I dodged that bullet temporarily.

Over the years with the aid of others, and by the grace of the Creator, I made it to that night in the hospital. Variously, I had found some excuses to keep going, but nothing profound enough to alter that long-standing mood. Since that night of a nose-to-nose choice, there have been only a few brief moments of wanting "out." I really did decide to live. It took almost dying to get me to accept being here in this life. And I found that reason. Such a price.

THIS IS A GOOD DAY

"We know what you've got . . . it's the bubonic plague!" Dr. Red sauntered in at day ten announcing the diagnosis as if he'd just found the cure for cancer. I was still in the ICU and had just stumbled out of the bathroom, dragging my lifelines and wound vacuum. *"What's so damn great about that?"* I thought.

"Wasn't that wiped out long ago?" I shot back at him. Not so, I was to learn. He said that the only accurate diagnosis for the plague is a blood culture test that takes 10 days to incubate. "How do you treat it?" I said in a squeaky voice.

"We have already been doing that with every antibiotic known to medicine."

I was so weak as I hobbled the five feet from the bathroom. It took every ounce of energy I had to make it to the much appreciated bed. My mind kicked in. It was not nearly as weak as my body. Just like the bunny, it keeps going and going. *"Where did I get that? Why had I not known it was still a cause of death, especially in New Mexico?"*

Within days my questions were answered when the Department of Health doctor came back to visit me. She asked permission to place traps on my property, believing the plague was hiding there aboard a rodent. I immediately developed a loathing for all creatures of their ilk, squirrels included, and I expanded my list to include rabbits, even after a week or so later when I got the report that no infectious agents were found. While she was talking to me, noise from the mini-vacuum cleaner attached to my arm caught her attention. She traced the tube to my upper left arm and asked about it. The drain tube under the large bandage was attached to an electrical suction source that had a low-level drone day and night. Plus I had to carry it and the rolling lifeline of IVs whenever I moved, which wasn't often. That site on my arm is where the doctors determined that the flea bit me, sending the deadly virus on its journey of death.

The arm wound was a consequence of a vigilant female doctor noticing the skin at that spot was not as soft as the surrounding tissue. That first week, through my barely conscious listening, I heard her say something about a biopsy. That was day five, a Friday. She took a tissue sample and sent it to a lab. On Monday she returned and told me that the sample had gotten lost. When she re-examined the spot, I heard that fateful, "Uh-oh." I knew that wasn't good. Immediately she scheduled me for surgery.

It happened the next day. The last thing I remember after being wheeled into the cutting room was asking the anesthetist his name. I awoke when it was dark, missing a chunk of arm the size of Rhode Island; and, man did it hurt. On top of other meds I was now receiving painkillers. Soon a technician arrived to explain the use of the "deep wound vacuum." Constant suction kept the bare tissue sanitary, except that the dressing covering it had to be changed every other day. Being a bit fog-bound, I was still able to ask about the skin that was re-growing "in there." "Won't that stick to the gauze?" He shrugged, as if to indicate that he was just the tech guy; and I should ask a higher-up. I would soon get the painful answer to my inquiry.

Two days later at about 8 a.m. a nurse arrived with a handful of painkillers. Two hours later the hurt-squad showed up to change the dressing. I almost couldn't stand it. A very compassionate nurse held my hand while another peeled off the white-turned-yellow pad—with new skin attached. There never were enough narcotics for that. From then on, my time revolved around getting ready for the pain, pain, then post-pain; not a pleasant cycle, at all.

A couple of friends found out about this torture. They scheduled themselves alternately to visit during the "event." They knew that I'd get crazy when given mind-altering drugs. I'd failed that test years earlier. The effects were still the same. The new prescriptions reminded my body and mind of those past times: sadness, guilt, shame, and, of course, fear. At one point two of my recovering friends were there, and I said to them, "I don't want to go back."

Their response still brings me a tear: "We won't let you." I believed them. They saved my life. So did the docs and right drugs. How many others never had the chance I was being given?

YODA VISITS

Lying there, wanting to move anywhere, not being able to, I squeaked out a simple prayer: "Help!" Soon after that, a barely audible tap-tap came from the ICU sliding door. Allowing the weight of my head to fall to the left, gravity took my eyes with it onto that slowly opening portal. Hobbling across the threshold was the last person I expected: old Carl Banks. The term "friend" would be a misnomer. As Yoda was something else to young Luke Skywalker, variously a nemesis or a mentor, so Carl was to me. Shuffling over to my bedside, he said, "Hey, what are you doing here?"

"What the hell's it look like?" I slurred.

"You don't look too well, I see. Think this is it? You gonna go Light Speed?" In my state of mind he could have been speaking Russian. "You know what I mean... stepping over to the other side? I've been there twice." That was his way of saying hello; he knew how to cut to the chase.

Every time we'd met over the last fifteen years, our conversations never lasted more than fifteen minutes each time, if that. Ten years and a couple of lifetimes older than I, he'd always been a man of few words. For certain, formality had never shown itself through him. I didn't know why, or the whole story, until that day.

"Carl, I can't say much; but I can listen to what you've got," I muttered with great effort.

He continued, almost as if he hadn't even heard me. "You may or may not want to hear this, but the Spirit tells me you need to. Few people know what I'm about to say. You're finally in a position to listen." He chuckled to himself as he took his right hand, slowly moved it, palm down, from left to right, indicating that I was laid out, incapacitated, and his captive audience. He was right, again. "Humility and knowing your right size is so important. I had to have it beaten into me on the chain gang in the South for twenty-eight months—then I got teachable. Are you teachable yet?"

In a quiet voice, lisping some as he spoke in broken tones, often considering his words, often not, sometimes just blurting out phrases, Carl continued. "Some of us had to get the message the real hard way. On that gang is where I learned to read and write, too, at age 30. Hell, my dad and older brothers beat me so bad I didn't talk 'til I was 3. By 11 I was a liar and a cheat, but mostly a thief. In-and-out of juvenile lockup, got trained by the best. Then at 18 it was prison or the Marines. I did not get locked up that time. They gave me an oral test 'cause I couldn't read. Semper Fi. Now that was hard-core training: no excuses, no surrender! Since I'd driven trucks on the streets of Denver for the Mafia boys, they stuck me behind the wheel where I stayed, in and out of Korea. After the war, back in the states, I ended up in Idaho writing bad checks in the bars. In those days bartenders were easy to fool. Finally, I got caught, ended up in a small-town jail, broke out with two other guys, knocking off the local armory on the way out of town in a stolen vehicle full of their weapons. When we sat around a campfire that night, it hit me what serious trouble I was in. 'Well, boys, I think we did it this time,' I said. 'And I know sure as hell there's a firefight comin', what with all the artillery we got—and I don't want to kill nobody. We better surrender ourselves.' They agreed, even liquored-up as we was. At sunup we drove off to a nearby town, walked into the police station and saw the deputy sittin' at his desk. When he asked what we wanted, I said, 'You know those three fellas who broke into the armory? We's them.' He started shaking so bad I had to dial his boss, the sheriff. I handed him the phone so he could say, 'Get over here, now!' We got his keys and put ourselves in a cell.

"When he got there that sheriff was kind to us, gave us coffee with our meal. Next day the Feds weren't so nice. They'd have worked us over if that boss man hadn't a-been there. Anyway, I did two years in a federal pen on an island in Puget Sound. That's where I met Rocky, who was the Mafia boss of the joint. He said I had a warped mind, but I couldn't fix that warped mind with the same warped mind. That made sense. It was my first message. He was hard on me 'cause he was doin' two life stretches and didn't want me doin' like he did.

"By the time I made parole I knew something had to change; but pretty quick I was drinkin' again, back to my old ways. Within a year I was stayin' in a mission in Milwaukee; I had some family there. Three-hots-and-a-cot plus clean clothes, that's what I needed then. Pastor Kelly, the reverend in charge, was the only man I could trust. One winter day–I remember 'cause it was cold and snowy–he pulled me aside, saying the FBI had been by looking for me. I had to find out for myself, so I went to the Post Office and sure enough my picture was there on the wall. You couldn't get more stupid than I was, or more alcoholic. Plus, I was really an angry guy, all right. Next day as I was going out of the warehouse sleeping dorm, the Feds were coming in. I didn't resist, for once. This time it was a weapons charge in Virginia."

It was as if Carl's voice was on volume control, and I could hear it in the background as I drifted in and out of consciousness. The more conscious, the louder it got. I'd never heard him talk so much. Ever.

"I knew I was going down for a while, but had no idea what was in store for me. To my surprise, the judge put me on a chain gang for only three years. That was a break, I thought. First day the captain got right in my face and said, 'Know what we do to Yankees here?'

" 'No, cap'n', I humbly said.

"In a slow southern drawl he whispered, 'We kill 'em!' My smart mouth almost went off, 'cept I knew he meant it. Within the week my hands and feet were bleeding from blisters. The other guys on the gang took care of me, even slowing the work down a bit. I got humbled, sure enuf. After a few months I got stronger, with Shorty from Mississippi doin' twenty years for armed robberies takin' care of me. He'd say, 'The harder the head, the bigger the hammer's needed to wake you up.'

"Brother Michael, you're layin' in that bed for a reason. I know you. You don't listen too well. You may think you're doin' OK, but Spirit told me to bring you this message. Mine came after twenty-eight months of hard labor when I got paroled back to that mission in Wisconsin. I wasn't the same guy. If I didn't do something different I was going back inside for life, a three-time loser. Spirit led me to a recovering fellowship, got me a hardcore Marine mentor who had been just like me. The principles on the path start with surrender. 'Not me!' I said.

"'A Marine will die first.' That's what he said I had to do: die to my old self. Then he led me on a path to Spirit. That was tough until he said, 'Carl, they call alcohol spirits for a reason.' Strange, I'd heard that myself from my first sponsor.

"It took me a while to pray, really askin' for help to change my ways. Next I had to do a thorough housecleaning of my past life and make restitution for wrongs. That was no fun, but I did it, and then I got off of parole that freed me to travel, so I went to San Diego. Of course I was lonely, so I got married. Not too smart, I can see now. It blew up in a year, but I didn't drink, hurt anybody, do a crime or go to jail. I figured I was healthy enough, so my new girlfriend, Becky, and I got married. That lasted a couple of years til we divorced, but no jail, again. I was learning something.

"Louie, my mentor at the time, said I needed to be alone, maybe in the desert. Off I went camping with hardly any stuff to the Colorado River area between California and Arizona for three months. While I was there, that first month an Indian Shaman showed up one morning for coffee. He said he saw me in a dream and was supposed to bring me a message. Just like you in that bed, I wondered, 'What the hell is this?' For so long I didn't think there was much hope for me. In a prison hospital they called me criminally insane. They were wrong. That Indian told me I was a carrier, a wounded healer with a message for so many others just as sick as me. Here's where you come in: you may not be as nuts or criminal as I was, Michael, but you are a carrier, too. I saw it in you years ago. Now I think you're ready, even lying there flat on your ass, hardly able to move." He laughed that wicked chuckle, like he got one over on me.

I smiled, eyes rolling in their sockets, and drifted off again. But I had heard him. Sure, carrier of what message?

LUPITA

She finally returned after what seemed like weeks; my sense of time was skewed. She had gone to help her daughter with the new grandbaby. "Señor, you look so much better," I heard, half-asleep, which was most of the time. Between staff taking vital signs of life each shift, daily blood draws, all kinds of tests, being the guinea pig for doctors' rounds, and visitors, rest was gotten in spurts and sleep was a premium in the hospital.

Because she was making noise as she fussed around the room, I came more to consciousness. Actually, Lupita's presence lit me up; and that voice—measured, melodic and peace invoking, beckoned me. She was the cleaning angel, much like Dr. Kubler Ross described in her book *On Death and Dying*. She was genuine and sincere. As she scurried about dusting and emptying the wastebasket, I listened to her family news, all the while waiting to ask about "him." At a moment when she stopped talking I quickly said, "You're the only person who seems to know about the Shadow."

"Sí," she said sheepishly, head down, inching nearer. "At the time I didn't think it was good to tell you. It was Señor Muerto-Death."

With a slight jerk of my head, hardly believing what I had heard, I said, "Really? Mr. Death?"

"He's around here a lot, but he didn't get you."

"You saw, I mean, see him a lot?"

"I try not to look, but mi madre told me to watch out years ago when I started working here. At first I was scared, then, it got OK after I prayed. That's what Mama told me to do. Something happened that took away my fears. He's just the guide into the next world."

"By that you mean he escorts you out of here?"

"Sí, when it's all over for you. Your life here isn't done yet. That's clear. We all have stuff to get done here. Do you know what you're supposed to finish?"

I was stunned. "You mean that I have something on this earth to complete?"

"Of course," she said quickly, just as shocked at my response as I'd been at hers. "Maybe this thing here was to get your attention, wake you up. I've seen it happen before to others."

She had my ears. Having been a licensed counselor in one on my many lifetimes, I knew how to listen when I had to. She was straight faced, seriously pointing to this major life event as an opportunity for change which is not something I've had a lot of grace with. It was about time, as I would later discover. She caused me to reflect.

THE JOURNEY

In my sixty years I had done so many things: traveled to foreign lands, worked at many jobs, walked the dark side, found the Light, loved, been loved, and now this! It'd been an interesting journey. "A long strange trip," a Dead-Head said. I started off life as a straight, Midwestern kid dropped into an Irish Catholic family. Though it was a safe place, fear showed itself, not unlike the way it does for most of us. Either a neighborhood bully was waiting to intimidate me, or brothers and sisters were snitching me off to Mom and Dad; it was present, right over there, always waiting.

Being the oldest I felt a responsibility to succeed. The first of twenty grandchildren to get a college education, I grew up helping others. It was trained into me as a guiding principle. After college, then marriage, I tried to be a professional helper. That lasted a few years until I heard the call west. The next phase involved construction, mechanics, bars, drugs and a look at the other side of life I'd only heard and read about. Then a ripping-my-heart-out divorce threw me into a single life I'd never really known before. A few years later, in my mid 30s, I moved to the southwest desert, hoping things would be better. When I got there, I arrived with all my same baggage. Back into the professional helping world I went. Licensure, community stature, and a home gave me some external worth. I just didn't feel it inside.

Next came a major change: no more drugs and alcohol. If you haven't tried that one, you're in for a ride. Abstinence provided me with a chance to look at my life from a totally different perspective, a spiritual one. I found a connection I'd always been searching for. But it wasn't easy. A self-searching personal inventory, making amends and willingness to change, these I recommend that you do not do alone.

Seven years later, in 1996, I went to work in Riyadh, Saudi Arabia at a substance abuse treatment center for Saudi men. That year was life altering. With few distractions, I did two things I had never made time for before: martial arts and writing. A Korean Master trained me so that when I left he said, "Michael is afraid of no one." Concurrently, I wrote over two hundred short essays. Leaving after a year's work, I began a seven-week walkabout back home to the USA.

Upon my return I just wasn't the same guy. Work began on my dream of building a mountain home. I transitioned out of the helping professions and became a full-time constructor. Three years later I landed in the hospital with Señor Muerto outside of my ICU door. Now, I was being told for a second time that I had something left to do in this life. OK, what is it? After what Lupita and Carl had told me, I knew I needed an answer.

SENOR MUERTO

There's only one way to say it: D-E-A-T-H. No one makes it out of here alive. Live long enough, and the idea of mortality makes itself known one way or another. Perhaps surviving a catastrophe brings the idea home. As a kid, the loss of a treasured pet evoked sadness and my parents explained that our dog Lady "went to doggie heaven." That was the best they had. Being Catholic, for us the end was Heaven, Hell or Purgatory. God made the final-decisions. And at that time we knew who He was. People with no mortal sins on their souls and no "temporal punishment" to work off went directly to Heaven. Those with smaller (venial) sins to account for or who had temporal punishment they had to face ("time they had to do") were sent to Purgatory until they were deemed ready to be released to Heaven. Those with mortal sins to account for—serious sins such as murder, adultery, missing Mass on Sunday and eating meat on Friday—went straight to Hell, no excuses allowed.

Then I heard, "Christ died for your sins." Poor Jesus hung on the cross for my lies, nastiness to younger siblings, and sexual longings. The mystery deepened. Man, I was a bad boy! How could a guy like me make it through the Pearly Gates? Surely, St. Peter had my name on the "**Do Not Admit**" list. In spite of this, I persevered through college and graduate school, thinking that redemption might lie in helping others. How close I was. But I began flirting with naturally induced spirits, alcohol and drugs. They connected me to the "other," but I always had to return to this mundane world of work, bills and other people's bullshit.

"Bulletproof" describes a kind of thinking phase I was in at the time. I did so many pushing-the-envelope crazy things for excitement and trying to experience life to its fullest. Little did I know or care how close to the stepping-off point I was. I'm not sure if they were attempts to live or die. Somewhere I read, "Life is like getting on a boat putting out to sea, which you know will sink." We all die . . . we just don't know when. Buddhists say to get prepared for the great letting go of our bodies by addressing attachments now. We've all got our hooks in this life, for sure; and the more we accumulate, the more we want to keep it, and fear death. Yet stepping over has its way of releasing us from all that's here; and it will do that, for sure.

My cleaning lady's description of the "shadow" made sense to me: he's just the Guide. The Grim Reaper has his own entrance at a hospital, especially in the ICUs and quarantine areas. Of all the rooms in all the hospitals, in all the world, he was camped outside of mine. It's true. Without antibiotic intervention, I would not have lived through my encounter with the bubonic plague. Yet I did.

Perhaps I am the voice of the millions of souls who did not. Each had a story, untold. My very first thought when I heard the diagnosis was how deeply I am connected to all of them. They died without telling their stories. I am still here to speak mine, and perhaps theirs.

Early on, when most frail from the onslaught, I vaguely recall a conversation about my passing out of this world. It was with Death. As best as I can remember, it went like this:

Michael (M): "Is it time for me to go? It feels like it. I can hardly move, walk or even lift a pen to sign an admit form."

Death (D): "I think I may have you. Your number has come up. Everyone's does, you know. Some think they can cheat me, but it's a momentary cheap thrill. I always win."

M: "True. But is there a determiner for when? Time's up! Time to go?"

D: "You two-legged beings always have to try and understand, don't you? Or make up reasons. You can do that if you want; but you have to realize there is impermanence to all of this. Everything comes and goes. It's not personal! You sound like

I've got something against you. It's just the way it is for all of life. I have nothing against you. All of your religions make up stories to give your life and passing some meaning. Believe me, I didn't have anything to do with setting up that plague thing. The Big Guy did that. I'm just doing my job, collecting spirits."

M: "You mean there is such a thing as a soul?"

D: "Put it this way: Your essence is you. It stays with you. Truthfully, you've been here before, past life stuff. I can't say much about it. That's all up to Her. Some essences seem familiar to me, like I've collected them before. But I can't really say. Now, let me see, your turn?"

M: "I hope not. That's a really dark corner there. No way. I don't want to go yet!"

D: "So you want to stay, now. I understand you haven't wanted to be there. Well, I have to check the reprieve list.... OK, I just got your ID cleared. Don't worry. I'll get you later. If it makes you feel any better about your life, use what's left for some useful purpose—help someone else! Talk to that cleaning lady. She's pretty sharp."

That's how it was on that dark early morning on day two or three. I'd been infected a week as *Yersinia Pestis* was making its murderous way through my bloodstream, killing every cell and organ it could. Then, the antibiotic showed up to rescue me. I wonder if The Creator had a hand in this? Recovering my health was not going to be easy. Losing so much muscle and body weight made even movement difficult. The most I could do was lie there, pray, and be the plague boy on the 4th floor.

However, a corner had been turned. I was still here. Now what?

RIYADH: ALLAH'S SAND BOX

There had been another "now what?" once, years before. Life had reached a "ho hum" spot where there wasn't much excitement. When I scanned the horizon of my life, it looked like the ocean from a sailboat when there is no wind. Then it just so happened that in the back of a professional magazine, I saw an ad for an employment opportunity as a training manager at an international hospital for the treatment of substance abuse. "Hmmmm. That sounds interesting." Off went my résumé to a post office box located in the United States. Months later, a call came crackling across the wires to the landline at my home. That was in 1994. Then I had a phone interview that sounded promising, and as my mind is wont to do, I assumed the job was mine. I was already packing. If my mind is not imagining a catastrophe, it's aggrandizing the positive aspects of a situation. Someone once called me an egomaniac with an inferiority complex, and there it was, right in front of my very eyes.

Returning to the mundane routine of everyday life was difficult, knowing adventure was just right there, over the horizon. At that time my professional life was cooking along with a small private practice office, delivering training programs, with contracts for Employee Assistance and the distraction of a Ms. Right, here and there. But focus was missing. It had been for years. This new job looked like an opportunity to fulfill my dream of combining world travel, work, and who-knows-what adventure. I kept anxiously waiting for that call to come, any day now. Finally, when I could take the suspense no longer, I called the 800 number, got to the right recruiter, then the news: they'd chosen someone else. A Scotsman had beaten me out. Of course I was discouraged, yet I found my way through it.

OK, what was the alternate adventure? In my city was a two-year vocational college that offered a degree in Construction Management. I enrolled. While working as a child abuse investigator

I studied all aspects of building science in the evenings. Many of my previous college courses could be applied to this degree, so I completed the degree requirements by taking specific classes in the trades.

Two years later, spring 1996, I got another call from that same recruiter. During this time their choice for Training Manager had done the job and was now headed back to Scotland. She asked me if I was still interested. It took all I had to keep from saying, "Are you kidding? I'm your man."

Of course, there was a process that included paperwork, the most complete physical I'd ever had, then the wait. Surprisingly, I got the good news only a couple of weeks after I'd submitted all the forms. In my mind I could hear myself say, *"Show me the airplane ticket!"*

If you've never put all of your goods in storage and packed a few things for a year's trip to the other side of the world, then you've got an experience coming. For a guy who had only been into Canadian and Mexican border towns, this was major. Places which I'd only heard or dreamed about now loomed near. But I'd never really used my passport, changed currency, tried to communicate to a non-native English speaker, or flown over an ocean. We all have to face things we've never done before; I just always seemed to have to do it alone.

A day or two after that phone call, I went to a recovery group meeting and when I was asked how I was doing, I spilled the beans. A member looked at me and said, "Michael, this is a gift from God. You go!"

The ticket arrived. Suddenly the adventure got very real. There was a lot to do: get a storage unit, pack what I wouldn't need, figure what I would need. How would I even know? What would I pack my belongings in for the trip? All I could think of was a large cardboard box. What was I thinking? No international traveler, as

I would come to find out, would do that. Airline baggage handlers are not nice to packages.

As the departure day loomed nearer, of course excitement shifted every now and then to fear. This was a real, no-kidding unknown. Isn't that what that visceral reaction is about:

F-E-A-R, or Future Events Appearing Real? We all know this one. It is hard-wired somewhere in the human brain, a survival mechanism. Except in this modern world, many of us mature adults (I was about to turn 50) base decisions on reality, not whether an adventure is connected to the saber-tooth tiger. Knowing that my take on reality might be a little skewed, having mentors outside of myself for double-checking decisions was essential.

Getting the thumbs-up from others, with appropriate safety checks, I proceeded to rent a storage unit, pare down my belongings, which included giving gifts to many people, then shaking my head at myself for keeping so many useless "treasures." All of my goods went into an 8 x 10 unit, neatly labeled, boxed, not to be seen for a year. I said goodbye to family pictures and childhood mementos, like that little cedar box from deceased Aunt Eleanor, or the holdable-in-two-hands brass lion from Father Butch. I wrapped them in old newspaper and gently placed them on top of the stack. Little did I realize this event was another letting-go. Somewhere I'd heard or read that courage is having fear, but going ahead anyway, which is what I was doing. .

Then there was the farewell to my sweetie at that time, Deb. We had met more than a year before at work, as child abuse investigators for the state children's protective services. Having the same birth sign, Leo, we had an immediate, innate affinity with one another. This seems to happen to most souls born under the same set of stars; either they are drawn together, or are really repulsed. Over the years I'd come to accept those parts of myself reflected by my sun-sign constellations: prideful—a group of lions, after all, is called a *pride*—outgoing, demonstrative, having a desire to help (if not control) and the inclination to be a leader. Deb, the lioness, also had some great sensuous mannerisms, like batting her eyelashes, a touch of a southern drawl, especially when she purred "Honeeee" drawn out to use up a whole breath—that melted me right away. Her Scarlett O'Hara charm had this Rhett Butler enthralled right off the bat. Even in casual work clothes her small female frame could sashay down the hallway and stop any traffic.

But as we talked, I discovered that she was just out of a marriage of twenty years. "No matter," I heard myself say. "We could both use some company." And within a month, after several flirtatious dates, we were a couple. God, we had fun. Again, my error was falling in love with someone who wasn't available. On top of that, delusion led me to ask her for some kind of commitment, including a year of celibacy while I was away. She laughed. I took it personally and withdrew, all the way to Saudi Arabia. I took it so hard, in fact, that my heart remained broken for months, even ten thousand miles away across an ocean in the middle of the desert.

Early on the Monday morning of my departure, my brother Dan, his wife and their kids Mark and Amy took me to the airport. All was going well until it was time to board the plane when final farewells were exchanged. Goodbyes have always been hard for me. This was no different. Mostly I kept my composure until I picked seven-year-old Amy up in my arms. We both began to cry. Since their births these children have been, well, just like mine.

Being their uncle, I was the on-call babysitter, diaper changer, wiper of tears, silly-hat wearer at birthday parties, godfather, witness to first bike rides, consoler for lost teeth, and congratulator for good grades. Now, it was time to leave them; and no one knew for how long.

Tears were in my eyes even as I put on the safety seatbelt. Sitting there, I relaxed for a bit. Then I knew there was one more phone call to make—to my mom in Ohio.

To say our relationship was contentious is an understatement. Her name was Ruth. I called her Ruthless, and she liked it when I joked that way. Since there were seven children, being the first, I got co-opted into caring for others at a very early age, as Mom was so busy tending to the youngest babies. It seemed to me I missed something. That something was maternal attention, and because I didn't get enough of it, I've tried to get attention in the world, especially from women. So, at some level, I had always resented her, though it's clear that she did her very best for all of us.

In the previous five years I had come to realize I had to manage conversations with her so as not to disclose too much of my personal life, as she had a wickedly dangerous tongue. Once, a couple of years before, I told her how I had a job, a home, a nice car and a girlfriend. Her response was, "It's about time!" That was it. At some point I realized she was incapable of having the loving mother-son interaction I craved.

I called her anyway. We spoke on the phone in New York between flights. She was excited for me. Over the years I sensed that she vicariously got excitement in her well-settled existence through me. Life without my father had been very hard on her for the two years since his passing. They had been joined at the hip for almost 50 years, though their lives had not been easy. We all missed him very much because he was such a good man. The oldest of five brothers who all made it safely home from WW II, he was a quiet guy who tried to be alone as much as he could, and was no doubt suffering from PTSD. He was well read and encouraged his offspring to get an education. Now I can say he was my hero.

At this point Mom suffered from diabetes that had taken her left leg, and had retired to a nursing home. She was feisty, opinionated about everything around her, and yet seemed unable to look inside herself; self-reflection was definitely not her forte. In spite of this, she wholeheartedly supported my trip, saying she knew that I had always wanted to travel the world. That was a surprise; I had never known that she understood that about me.

So it was on this last phone call, just as I was about to leave, we had the conversation I had always wanted to have with her. For once she was kind and loving. That was the best sendoff I could have asked for. After that I wrote her weekly. Our mother/son relationship had changed for good. I boarded the plane feeling lighter.

Flying across the ocean is an experience not to be missed in this lifetime. Boredom is in the seat next to you. (It's not unlike lying in a bed in an ICU, pretty much unable to move.) Spending twenty hours in a flying box forces you to examine your use of time, if nothing else. Take a good book, be ready to talk to strangers, bring a portable music device, but most of all prepare to deal with time alone. (Hemingway is reputed to have said, "The cure for loneliness is to be alone." Well, he killed himself when he was not allowed to return to his beloved Cuba . . . so much for that advice.)

Thankfully the 747 was not full. Seasoned travelers did what they had seen done before. Claiming the three seats on one of the outside aisles, they lifted the armrests, threw a blanket over themselves, and started the journey with a space-claiming nap. It was about noon when the trip began. Because we were headed east, daylight accompanied us for a few hours, with clouds over the blue Atlantic as the only scenery outside of the windows. Since there were plenty of empty seats, I felt free to move around when the Fasten Seat Belt sign was off. Cruising the aisle as I returned to the seat I'd staked as my claim, I saw a young man, perhaps Arabic, sitting alone looking ready for a conversation. At some level, my intuition told me that a conversation with him would likely be mutually beneficial. "Mind if I sit down for a moment?"

"No, not at all," he responded in perfect British-accented English, smiling as he pointed to the vacant aisle seat. Next, he stuck out his right hand to open the exchange, saying, "My name is Khalid, what's yours?"

"Michael, and I'm headed to Riyadh for the first time."

Giving me a two-second appraisal, he surmised, "Well, you're on an adventure, and I'll bet it's not to do a pilgrimage to Mecca."

"Correct you are. Actually, I'm taking a job at Al-Amal Hospital for the Ministry of Health."

"That's the facility where my countrymen go to deal with addictions, isn't it?" he asked.

Without much thought I concluded that he was educated, from a family with money, perhaps with Royal connections, and a modicum of compassion for those suffering.

"Perhaps you know that we have quite a problem in that area. It can be embarrassing to families to have a member who insults the clan with inappropriate behavior. Allah prefers respect for our bodies, each other, and the world we live in. I am pleased you are coming to assist us."

What a welcome, when I hadn't even set foot on Saudi soil, yet. "Thanks, how kind of you," I said. "A country that focuses on prayer and honorable ways must be spiritual, for sure."

With both elbows on either armrest, hands under his chin, head nodding slowly, through a smile he said, "Well, maybe. I think we probably need to pray five times a day just to keep us focused. Make no mistake, all aspects of the human condition are present there. I've been studying medicine at Harvard and now I'm going home to practice, and I have seen the best and the worst in the States. We are no different. There will be many lessons for you in your stay. Do not judge us too harshly. Keep an open mind to our humanity and you will do OK. You will have respect as you give it." Just then the captain bid all passengers to return to their seats for dinner service. We bowed to each other, exchanging thanks as I stood up to leave. Then he took my right hand in his, gazed intently in my eyes, and said, "Allah be with you, my friend." Interactions between strangers can go any which way. This one was permeated with a kindly welcome, an injunction that suggested I mind my Ps and Qs, but was a great start to my adventure. As I ate the five-star airplane meal, anticipation overcame the fear and even a touch of excitement arrived with the dessert. The adventure was afoot.

Several months after my arrival I learned that Khalid was a minor prince in the royal family, who purposely greased the wheels for me at the hospital with indigenous administrators. As I discovered, that's how things worked there: not so much what one knew, but the quality of relationships and "heart" that one brought.

But now my orientation to Saudi Arabia began at the country's main airport, which was designed to resemble a series of large tents. I made my way slowly through that enchanting building. It was a good thing that I didn't have to pay much attention to where I was walking, for I acted like a gawking tourist. Military personnel with automatic weapons stationed every couple of hundred feet or so got my attention. However, having a low threshold of amazement can be a double-edged scimitar. All of the newness enchanted me. Being in a genuine state of wonder served me well, because it dispelled the impression that many Saudis had of Americans as know-it-alls.

At the Customs desk, I saw that the large cardboard box holding my goods had all but disintegrated. Buried in it was a copy of the Koran in English and Arabic that I had gotten at a used bookstore in New Mexico. The official smiled at me; it turned out to be a good luck charm.

I passed the Customs inspection, which checked for contraband such as Christian material or anything Jewish or Buddhist-related. That was my first lesson in what a theocracy is like. Islam is everywhere; and Saudi Arabia is not a tourist destination. Unless a visitor comes for a religious purpose or to visit family, he must obtain a sponsor, and must surrender his passport. Of course, military are exempt, as well as diplomats. All others, including me, got a replacement I.D. that designated religious affiliation. Somehow everyone agreed that my picture looked very Arabic.

An affable driver loaded my bags and my tattered box into the limousine, driving me directly to Al-Amal Hospital. Arriving dressed in Levi pants, casual shirt and cowboy boots, I was immediately summoned to the auditorium for the hospital staff meeting. Gulp! Little did I know I was the guest of Honor. First impressions in that world tend to last forever, as I discovered over the course of time, and, thankfully, I was able to control my sometimes-undisciplined tongue. World public opinion is mostly not favorable toward my nationality. *The Ugly American* is more than a great old movie; it tells how people from other countries are likely to perceive us. As I was standing there in front of a hundred men from 20 countries, I was humbled. By nature I am kind and deferring, reserving my smart-alec nature until I feel comfortable in the crowd. That took a while, as I really needed to get the lay of this land, lest someone took offense and I found myself out of there on the next flight. That really could have happened. To my credit, about halfway through my tour of duty I was informed that I did not seem like the normal American. Most of those who said that had never met one.

The afternoon after my arrival my boss, Joe, an American hospital administrator hired to advise, sat me down for a Dutch-uncle chat about how things really worked in this world. He recommended that I take the "You are a guest here" approach, which I did, because I was.

After my grand entrance, I was finally taken to my living quarters in an apartment complex that housed people of several nationalities who worked at our facility. Doctors from India, nurses from the Pacific Rim, an engineer from the Philippines and housekeeping staff from Africa were all thrown together. A guard at the entrance gate was supposed to keep intruders out; but I heard that they also monitored closely who and what entered and the goings-on that occurred inside. No immoral shenanigans allowed. Early on I decided to play by the rules, though I was to learn that Westerners were cut some slack. To some degree they could get by with behavior that was not tolerated in Saudis.

My flat was spacious compared to many others. The translator assigned to me, Mohsen, an Egyptian, commented later upon seeing my place that his wife, kids, uncles, aunts and their kids could all live in the space allotted to me. Many third-world residents have said that they would like to come back to this life as a pet in an American household. Experiences there led me to see the impact cultural idiosyncrasies have on us all.

It was the praying five times a day that got my attention more than anything else. Just like clockwork, when the call to prayer started, everything else stopped: businesses closed, traffic came to a standstill, and religious police questioned pedestrians. That was just the way it was, and taken for granted.

Well into my stay I was swimming in our pool daily, hanging out with the Brits, writing nightly about my experiences, and taking martial arts training from a Korean master not unlike Mr. Miagi. At 50 I felt like the Karate Kid.

Having my recovering fellowship already established there gave me untold opportunities with well-traveled expatriates. They took me to places I never could have found on my own, including chop-chop square where corporal punishment was administered. That type of punishment was the accepted way of keeping the peace, and it seemed to work. On one of my trips to the *souks*, a specialized market, I saw amazing gold jewelry. My four sisters received 24-carat gold earrings that I purchased there.

About two-thirds of the way through the year, I realized that I did not want to stay any longer than I had to, for I found the atmosphere too repressive. When I had been there ten months, I was informed that I would receive thirty days of vacation if I stayed the entire year. I left after 11 months.

I exchanged my one-way airfare home for an around-the-world trip so I could make stops here and there as I journeyed westward. Thanks to my Egyptian friend and translator, Mohsen, I was granted special "brotherhood" with the Egyptians, and my friend Dr. Vincent from the hospital connected me to the Indian community. I was well cared for.

With my six-week walk-about looming near, I had a soulful chat with Mohsen. We talked about the Creator, whom Muslims must call Allah. Once I said, "Yae, God!" He smiled and said, "We say Ya, Allah!"

It seemed to me that in a culture in which everyone prayed five times a day, people would act more spiritual than I found most of them to be. "Just because we are so religiously regulated does not guarantee anything, Mr. Michael. We are human, too," explained Mohsen. "Do not think ill of us, as we are creatures subject to our common humanity."

He knew my birth sign was Leo. As I was tearfully leaving, he called me *Asad Allah*. That, as I discovered, means "Lion of God."

In that plague recovery bed years later, hardly able to move, all I could do was squeak like a kitten, and pray for help. Memories washed over me as I quietly lay there healing from an international killer who had taken-up residence in New Mexico and me.

SPIRIT REP COMES A-CALLIN'

On a quiet day as I was resting between blood draws, as well as being the day's item for intern inspection, a knock came at the door. "Hello, I'm the chaplain, may I come in?"

"Sure, I'd like someone to pray with," I said. After the usual amenities like, *"What are you here for? Oh, that's terrible. Are you a Christian?"* (most chaplains are Bible-based folk), she started the prayer. Almost always I felt tears well up during this part. There was so much shared compassion and intention to connect with Spirit; it touched me deeply. (Of course my emotions were raw–a brush with death will do that.) Even though the names for her god were different from mine, I didn't care. They're all the same to me. At "Amen" my eyes were wet. . Never during this tribulation was I ever angry with the Creator. I didn't understand why this had happened to me, but I wasn't angry.

In this medical cloister I was in, I was very sensitive to kindnesses. This time was no different. But the Reverend Lady did something different after praying. She asked me about my life. In about fifteen minutes I thumbnail sketched it out pretty plainly, including the transformations. By the end she was moved, I know. She was in tears, too. We became connected. That wasn't the only time I shared prayers. With most of my visitors, we ended our time together holding hands in a moment of thoughtful acknowledgement of the Creative Intelligence. That brought me a lot of comfort.

My mentor, Keith, was always there. Our very first meeting, years earlier, was over a prayer. At that time I asked him a question that puzzled him. He said he had no response, except to pray about it, together. He taught me that...such a lesson. Back in the ICU when I started to heal, he told me that initially he had thought I was a goner. My weakness, delirium, plus the bad reaction to a drug all led him to believe that death was imminent. I believed that too.

When it became clear that I was going to live, fewer visitors came and their visits became less frequent. He said that it was because they knew I was going to live. But three people kept coming: my brother Dan, Keith, and Bubba—all prayerful men connected to Spirit. None are holy-holy pious kinds. They're guys who live honorably and love me. Most of the time I felt strange just lying there motionless and receiving guests. Once a good friend gave me a foot massage, and shaved me—I'd never had that done before. By allowing him to give to me I know at some level he received as well. People made all the difference.

Among those who made a difference were a couple named Mark and Sonja. Earlier that year I'd met them when there were newly arrived in New Mexico from Arizona. They reappeared at just the right time one morning when I couldn't eat the conventional breakfast in the ICU. In fact I vomited when I saw and smelled the usually good fare. Keith tried hard to get me to eat, for I had actually lost 25 percent of my body weight by then. Mark and Sonja are into health food; they eat what I call "nuts and twigs." They saw my difficulty, went to a store and got me yogurt and fruit. That changed my diet from then on.

Not having any "real" food—donuts, hamburgers, sodas or good coffee—left me craving, especially after day ten. Dan brought me a good burger and a cup of great coffee, but my appetite was so bad that I barely touched them. That was real kindness. It was everywhere. Being a "giver," I didn't realize that I had not learned how to be a "receiver." But here, in this situation, I could not help but experience being loved. So, in the middle of tragedy I got to be taken care of.

Not everyone survives the plague. There's a less than a 50-50 chance of survival without medication, if the disease is discovered in time. (The Centers for Disease Control say that 1 in 14 who are infected die here, in the USA. Rubbish!). I survived, and I attribute that to modern medicine and the interventions of others, including their prayers. At some time in my past I had read books that showed the positive effects of conscious quiet communication with the Other. Enough of that inquiry has stayed with me such that I believe it works; but a tad bit of doubt remains on my part. Good thing my friends believed it and shot good 'vibes' my way. Something (antibiotics?) and/or Someone interceded (my brother/doctors) so I began to heal. Perhaps the Creator uses people, places, things and situations to make the difference.

Pretty much we humans are "fox-hole" pray-ers. We pray only when we're desperate, and our prayer consists of something like "Get me out-of-this, and I'll...." Over the course of the years before this life crisis I had formed the habit of praying every day. My parents as practicing Catholics had set that example. Perhaps I inherited it, also; more likely I was driven to it by drug and alcohol addiction. Where it came from does not matter. Every day I ask for: health, wealth, happiness, love, peace, fun, safety and a sense of Your Presence for all of my family. I name them one by one, and see their faces. All of my brothers and sisters are well, and nieces have delivered babies safely. No one has been in jail. They're happy. I'm alive. Prayer has had something to do with this, I know.

After asking for blessings for family, I call to mind those suffering: children being abused or institutionalized, the parentless and homeless, those dying or those who have been told they are going to die soon, veterans, war victims and their families, people paralyzed, single heads of families, pregnant women, normal folks raising kids, leaders (especially religious), alcoholics, junkies, those incarcerated and thieves. Nobody prays for thieves. Everybody has been stolen from and hates a thief. So do I. Except the last time I was ripped off, I couldn't stand my own anger, so I undertook a prayer project for the thieves. I got over my anger. So, it wasn't like

I was prayer-less when I was stricken with this illness. Not, I'm sure, unlike the millions of others who have died of the plague and prayed. I just got drugs and another wake-up call, as Lupita pointed out. But why me?

TATS I'VE KNOWN

"Where'd you get that ink?" I blurted out as he entered the room. He was not too tall, maybe 5 ft. 10, but the stocky frame that carried him seemed well conditioned...he was a guy not to be trifled with. But he was smilingly humming a tune. In the middle of a jaunty step when he heard my question, he stopped. Empty glass blood vials rattled as he abruptly turned toward me.

"What'd you say? Are you talking to me?" That tone, along with a stance that indicated he was somewhat offended, was too practiced to be accidental; it was probably the result of hours spent in front of a mirror trying to emulate a infamous Robert DiNero line.

"Yea, of course I am. Nobody here but us guys; and you're the one with those well done tattoos, right?" He didn't quite know how to take my response. I knew he was thinking, Who would be talking to me this way, especially in a hospital?

Slowly, with a bit of a swagger, he approached the voice that had verbally assaulted him.

"What's a mouth like that, on a guy like you, doing in a bed like this?"

Quickly the voice shot back, "For once, you blood suckers are talking to the body you stick your needles into. Mostly your brothers and sisters slither in, poke me, grab the vital bodily fluid, then poof! Gone without a 'how-do-you-do.' At least I got your attention. "True", said Mr. Painted Body. "Not a lot of patients talk to me, which is just as well. I'm here to do a job, not chat my way through the day. So what's your story, anyway?"

"Oh, mine's just the bubonic plague, been here a month, lost 40 pounds, relearning to walk, not sure when I'll get out of here or what I'll do when I do." He jerked his head. "I thought that was gone, like in the Middle Ages or something. Too bad, at least it looks like you'll make it. It hasn't affected your mouth any I see. You'd be surprised how many don't make it, not from the plague. You're the first person I've ever met who's had it. I mean other people I draw blood from, then the next day, gone." "Yep, could have been me, for sure, "I said. "Now it's my turn. What's a guy with tats like you got–well done, by the way–doing in the blood trade?"

He thought for a moment, then said, "My family was in medicine, but I didn't want to live my life, their way. Mostly nobody does" I said, "but one way or the other we really play out the family script, don't we? We don't do it their way–we do it our way–except it comes out looking a lot like them. We can't help it. They're our teachers. Not a surprise that parents live on through us, like it or not." Just like me, I'm sure, my dad watched over his brothers as best he could. Lou, his father, was an alcoholic, which left scars on my father's little soul. Dad was a quiet but thoughtful man, troubled by anxiety, worry, and depression. He took meds. Life never seemed to be enough; nor was he for it, it seemed to me. He raised seven healthy, law-abiding children, had thirteen happy little grandchildren, most with college degrees (one Ph.D., one lawyer, several master's degrees). While he was alive I felt like I didn't live up to his idea of an oldest son; most children don't. Being raised mostly by my mom in his emotional absence, I really ended up more like her: affable, opinionated, emotionally volatile, and righteous about how others (and life) should be, but spiritually oriented. Both of them were that! Helping others has been a guiding principle for me, like them. Yes sir, my family is who I am, plus a few characteristics I've thrown in for good measure. Just like you, tattoo boy."

"True" he said. "This is really weird; to be talking to a patient in the hospital about my personal life. You're kind of like a bartender that a drunk talks to, except this isn't a bar." After a moment, during which he was deciding if he wanted to deepen this inquiry, he said, "My family wanted good things for me, but my mom died when I was a kid, then my doctor dad fell apart, so my older sisters raised me. They were nurses. It's in the blood, right? There's a connection I never saw before. Better get on with my job, man. Raise your arm." Despite 50 previous blood draws, he found a vein, took a couple of small tubes of my life's liquid, thanked me then vanished.

As he left me alone with nothing but that wandering mind, memories of others who wore tattoos floated onto the screen. Since a lot of my professional life had been spent in mental hospitals, jails, and prisons and around people who abused substance, tattoos were commonplace. They do seem to show up in a different population than doctors and lawyers and other professional people. One of the first guys I met twenty years earlier who looked like he'd been steeped in color was Tommie, a world-class boxer, raised in "the hood" He was about 5 ft. 4 and spoke softly, but his fists were his big sticks in the ring. He told me in confidence that he could do all right for a while, but queen Chiva (heroin) almost always brought him down, back into rehab. "It's not the quitting, it's the staying quit that's the problem." In his treatment center room he took off his shirt, turned around and showed me his bare back, to which I could only respond, "Wow!" There inscribed was a beautiful replication worthy of exhibition in a museum. The multicolored image of the Christian Madonna, her arms outstretched, adorned with a halo, stars and beauty the likes of which I'd never seen, were in front of me. Most religions have a female representation like this. Being familiar with the icon did not keep me from staring at the exceptional detail with amazement. I was overwhelmed. When he started to move after a few minutes, I stopped him and asked if I could take more time to study the picture. He allowed it. Part of me was moved enough to shake my head in wonder at the work of art. "Man, that's beautiful. Where'd you get it?" I asked.

My primo (cousin) does great work, no? Almost all of my stuff is from him," he said.

Pride filled his body when he straightened his shoulders, making a long slow loop with his head to a grinding and popping sound, which he seemed to relish. Ripples in his upper body musculature became visible as he pulled his arms together in front of his torso, expanding the Lady on his back. Obviously he'd done this before, no doubt in a boxing ring under lights before a cheering crowd. Looking at him, eyes closed, head back, it was as if he were right there listening to the announcer, "In this corner... Tommie the Mexican Mauler under the Protection of the Lady herself, undefeated in 30 fights...."

However, not even the Blessed Mother could save him from the unholy bitch, heroin.

She'd kicked his ass on and off for twenty years; and just when he thought he had her on the ropes, she spun him around and he went down for the count. Several rehabs, arrests, loss of his world title and overdoses beat him so badly that he didn't have enough heart to answer the bell one morning. It had all caught up with him. Or maybe a stroke took him out in the middle rounds of his life. I was sad when I got the news.

Just before I met The Boxer, his counselor Huey, came into my life. Actually we met when I was an instructor for a new University Extension program in substance Abuse. During a Practicum class in Roswell I noticed him, sitting in the back of the room, quiet, watching me with hawk eyes as I led the class. It was an evaluation that did not evoke fear, as many others had. On a break I discovered that twenty years earlier he had been a sniper in the Vietnam War. Damned assassins, always looking for the perfect moment to take that one killer shot. He did. The following day, Saturday, after the class he invited me to a recovery roundup meeting at which a fellow from Texas, Jim, was speaking.

My acceptance of that invitation changed my life. To my surprise several hundred folks filled the hall next door. After a brief introduction featuring readings, which let me know I was in a recovery meeting, Jim was introduced. Right off the bat he started telling his story, which everyone around me found humorous. I didn't. How could these people be laughing at the tragedy he reported as a result of drinking: lost jobs, marriages, hospitalizations, bankruptcy; all told with a straight face, almost as if the story was a mystery to him as well. Then he relayed what it was like now that he was abstinent, following a spiritual path that included carrying a message of hope to others whose lives were also so afflicted. There are those moments when one is brought up short by the leash of life, coming nose-to-nose with the Truth; which, by the way, he said would set me free, not without first causing me pain and pissing me off. It did that, plus more. A thinly veiled dark place in me became lit like a large neon sign: YOU GOTTA DEAL WITH THIS, NOW!

Talking (and listening) to others after the gathering, I heard stories that were true of my life also. Weird how that works when one's ears are finally open to hear that which wasn't allowed in before. There comes a time when it's impossible not to listen. As a licensed substance abuse counselor, educated and trained, there was not much new in that field that anyone could tell me that I hadn't already encountered. Bottom line: I was incapable of applying myself to the information. But sitting in that large room with those folks, the volume on my defensive mind chatter diminished; and what that speaker said got through whatever barrier(s) had been erected. By some indistinguishable process, the mind that drives the bus of this body had gotten programmed: "No need to apply this stuff to your life!"

Subtle forces shape our thinking. Clearly, our culture, parental influences, family constellation (birth order), religion, in my case Catholicism, education, aspirations, being male, Caucasian, flavoring of alcohol dependence all conspired to insulate me from really learning about myself. Early on, guilt as well as shame were mechanisms used on me which I internalized to later manage my own behaviors. Since I was not a big fan of pain or its cousin, suffering, avoiding feeling bad about myself meant excluding information that would contribute to self-examination. Some use the term "denial" to label refusals to admit to a reality others easily acknowledge.

A teacher once said, "If one person calls you a horse's ass, forget it. If two people do, then go get fitted for a saddle." Ignore-ance has something to do with control issues, for sure; but real-I-zations are difficult to discount, especially when one is ganged upon by them. Coincidentally, when there's just too damned much dissonance between reality and what I've been telling myself about it, I know something's got to change. One option is that I just might have to admit that perhaps I may be wrong about something, like there's a chance that my assessment about things might not always be right. Finally I was able to hear, and admit that alcohol consumption was affecting my thinking and acting more than I realized. I was beginning to consider that what others were saying about their lives had implications for me. If what they were saying about their lives was true for me, then I may be like them. The opening occurred after a crisis, then a willingness, then conversation.

We talk ourselves into living the way we do, or don't. Perhaps the choice of a path we take is not always at the level of a conscious conversation with ourselves; but that doesn't mean there isn't a discussion or a talking back-and-forth rattling around in our heads. The first time I heard it I had to sit quietly in a noiseless place; then listen. By golly, I noticed "it." Such a revelation I had. You mean all of that noise has been going on and I didn't even know it? Yes, Michael, I'm afraid it's true. Your life is a product of all that that mind has directed you to do, which is as far as possible to avoid feeling icky and go for what feels good. That's just how people are. We all try to make good lives for ourselves with bewilderment, frustration, terror and despair living right below the surface.

So, at 42 I awakened. Quitting alcohol was long overdue. But really, why had it taken so many years? Probably it had to do with the business as usual aspect of my day-to-day life. Mostly habituated existence, without any significant modifiers, allowed it. Things continue. Just like a law of physics: life goes on and on in this petty pace until something or somebody interrupts the flow. That's one of the requirements for change. There has to be a significant need for things to be different.

Even our brains are wired that way. Patterns of electrical energy follow least resistant pathways. These neurotransmitter byways get developed over time, really controlling our lives. What's usual and normal is what we've done before that worked out OK. Benefits came to us from acting a certain way, even if that way was short sighted. Not seeing the bigger picture with all of the possible factors did not stop the consequences. Some whose programming includes looking at the larger scene of life with all its vagaries, were not able to see the trees for the forest. Ways of acting, perceiving, even thinking, have been pretty well crystallized by the teenage years. So strong are the electronic freeways in our noggins that we invent (manufacture) reasons (excuses) to justify our actions and do not see or accept realities in front of us. Nobody wants to admit to being programmed; but without significant influence our lives play-out as scheduled. So where's the choice in all of this?

Someone described choice as "after consideration, picking." For the most part consideration rarely enters into the process, especially where abuse of alcohol or drugs is concerned. Given where and how, in the brain, they have an impact, substances often do the deciding.

A man takes a drink.

The drink takes the drink.

The drink takes the man.

That's not always what happens, but it's something to be wary of. It took a full year of abstinence for me to become comfortable with that life style. Little did I realize how such a seemingly insignificant aspect of my life had become such a major player in it. I had become inured to my own life.

Then there's the frog story. A frog is in a pan of water on the stove with the heat on. It's a story, after all, so we don't know exactly how he got there. Somebody comes along and turns up the burner under poor froggie's pan. Since he can adjust his body temperature to his environment, he does so, until he's cooked. He altered himself until his surroundings got him. If only he'd looked over the side of the pan he might have noticed that this didn't look good for him. Or if only he'd had a friend to point out the peril. Apparently there is a limit to a frog's inquiry, as was the case with me.

I am going to schedule an appointment at Mom's Tattoo Parlor when I get out of here.

When I called and talked to the artist he said he could put a nice frog on the back of my right hand just below the fingers with a caption: YOU'RE JUST LIKE ME.

FINDING OUT MORE ABOUT THE PLAGUE

"That can't be—didn't it go away in the Middle Ages?" I said incredulously. Not so, Michael. After the official diagnosis was made, I was driven to find out more about this disease. Brother Dan brought me materials. To just hold a book was a challenge, given my weakness. Concentrating was out of the question, so pen and pad replaced ability to focus: anything I read of importance had to be written down to be remembered. There's an adequate supply of academic material about plague, and historical fiction about it abounds. There are eyewitness accounts in journals, strange as it might seem. In the 14th century a retired military officer came into the King's employ as a logistics man providing food to naval ships. He kept a daily, detailed log during the Great Plague.[1] Even fictional stories about documented circumstances are an interesting read.[2] There have been several films based on circumstances of the times.[2] But one has to have a real personal or academic interest to get to know about the other two pandemics and various epidemics, which have afflicted mankind. And there are few written first-person account of surviving this torment.

History is amazing. It is not like solving a complex math problem, or a physics puzzle that opens new vistas. I do not know why, but since taking an upper-level college history class, what has occurred before us interests me so much. Now I'm especially interested in learning about the disease that brought me to the brink of death.

For all of my educational life, history was about facts: "On a certain date such-and-such happened." When I first started to examine the facts of the plague, it was like that. As I learned about many contributing events, it became obvious that dates were only markers. One event can have any number of antecedents. Any accident occurs that way. For example, the Challenger disaster was attributed to an inadequate "O" ring. But that flawed piece of rubber got there through a series of happenings. More like the result of a chain reaction that culminated in the catastrophe. Seemingly unconnected events, like a volcano on the other side of the earth, can generate an effect halfway around the world. Changes in weather such as seasonal variations in rainfall, earthquakes, massive fires, and alteration of trade routes all collaborated to create conditions for the first pandemic of plague around 600 A.D. Receiving its name, Justinian's, from the Roman emperor at that time, it killed tens of millions. It was not confined to a small area, either. The Roman Empire stretched from Lebanon to Scotland, Vienna into North Africa, then from Paris to the southern border of Egypt. The population had reached 50 million by 250 A.D. Then the biomedical happened: smallpox and gonorrhea from A.D. 250 to A.D. 450, followed by plague until 640 A.D. or so. That civilization, based on manpower not machinery, was decimated. A quarter of the population was gone—more than 12 million, just like that. Who would grow the food, exchange the goods, or protect the borders from invaders? With a smaller tax base and fewer funds for the military, the Empire could not protect its undefended frontiers, which now were ripe for barbarian invasions. That happened. One academic source suggests that the "other-worldliness" of Christianity may have diverted attention from more critical matters.[3] Certainly the threat that science posed to the Church's authority inhibited development of medical breakthroughs. Faith healing was the intervention of choice for the disease. Historians conclude that the rat-borne march of death lasted until 750 A.D. in 8- to 12-year cycles.

By 700 A.D. all of the eastern and southern shores of the Mediterranean were ruled by Arabic-speaking Muslim lords. Even Turkey had come under Arab rule.[4] The first year of the Muslim calendar is 623 AD, coincidently. There is discussion in some of the literature on plague that Muslims, like the Christians, resorted to "other-worldly" healing options that did not facilitate dealing with day-to-day crises, and may in fact have inhibited scientific and medical advancement. Islam was in Jihad at that time, motivated by religious fervor. Any death was considered martyrdom worthy of reward in the next life.

When I tell someone that I was in the hospital dying from bubonic plague, their usual response is, "I thought that was gone with the Middle Ages." Well, I asked that question, too. But it's not so at all. The Black Death is just the one we've heard the most about. There actually have been two other major waves of death attributed to plague, as well as other significant epidemic outbreaks as recently as the one in 1994 in India.

The First Book of Samuel, Chapter 5, Verse 9 says, "The Lord's hand was against that city, throwing it into great panic. He afflicted the people of the city, both young and old, with an outbreak of tumors in the groin." I have my "mark of the beast," as well. The scar is located on the inside of my upper left thigh. Technically, what happens is that a hemorrhage occurs at places termed DIC: Disseminated Intravascular Coagulation.

The first strike by the plague was followed by about a 600-year hiatus. There seems to be no scientific explanation for this. However, there is incontrovertible evidence about the second.

---

1. Moote, L. and Moote, D.; Extensive diary of military provisions officer.

2. Long, R.E. (1994).Ingmar Bergman, film and stage.1957 Ingmar Bergman film, *The Seven Seals* about Plague in 14th. Century Sweden.

3. Rosen, W. Justinian's Flea. Map of Roman Empire 305-565 C.E.

4. Ibid. Extent of Arab rule by 700

AD 1348

People living in plague-ravaged communities could not understand why this calamity had befallen them. Imagine a conversation between a man and his parish priest, whom he is hoping will provide answers.

"Father, what is happening here? Our two babies have died, my sons are sick and my wife is so worn out from taking care of everybody. Neighbors are dead. On my way to the fields yesterday I waved at one. He was dead when I passed on the way home. Some of my friends have just disappeared–I don't know where they went. No one has ever seen anything like this before. The piles of corpses are everywhere. There's no place to escape the stench of rotting flesh. That smell is horrible. There are more to bury than those of us left to do it. Dogs, rats and other animals are eating on those thrown into the streets. Nobody knows what to do.

"I know you are praying for us, and preaching that we're sinners who need to repent. God is really angry at us, I guess. But my family and me have not done anything wrong. We pray, go to Mass, try to help others–what else can we do? Those "star-people," astrologers, say it's the fates–nothing anybody can do. Sure seems true. Margaret and I lie in our straw bed at night. She cries. I try to be strong, but I'm scared. Those herb people came in their funny costumes, cut on my little girl to bleed the evil humors out. She still died–and I couldn't help her. That hurt so much. Why would God let that happen? I almost went out of my mind. Word has come that this is some kind of plague. Those of us left try to keep foreigners out of our village–maybe they're carrying it. People are running away, I guess.

"There is so much pain–all we can hear is screaming, day and night from the sick ones and their families. All we can do is pray, avoid others...and cry when our babies died. First they stopped playing, then wouldn't get up, wouldn't eat, went limp in our arms. One of us held them close while the other tried to coax food into their little mouths. (There's not much on the table since the farmers are gone, too). After a day or two, red blisters came out onto their skin; next those sores turned purple, then black. Not long after that our babies passed on, right in our arms. Burying them was the hardest. Who wants to put your flesh-and-blood in the ground, cover them with dirt, say goodbye, then walk away?

"Why them and not me? They never hurt anybody. Please don't say that it's just the will of God. It's not right. Their names got added to the List of Mortality, posted by the village leaders, who can't do anything else, anyway. I've got to get us out of here. Margaret's sister lives a couple of villages over, deeper in the woods. We'll be safer there, I'm sure. This can't last that long."

THE NEXT ONE

The last real outbreak of plague started in China around the end of the 19th century. It migrated to India, Hawaii, then on to the United States. Aboard ships, death made its way east through the Pacific Rim. Hitching a ride on a ship to Hawaii, Chinatown was eventually burned in an effort to stop the deaths. In January 1900 the bacillus landed on our shores

The plague found a home in San Francisco. Of course the good leaders of the city commenced a vigorous program of denial. Nobody seemed to want to admit "**It's here!**" Public Health doctors in 1900 knew what was attacking. In 1894, Alexandre Yersin, who had studied with Louis Pasteur, eventually identified the bacillus in Hong Kong. Plague was discovered to be carried by rats. There is a wonderful book written about this poor, one-man crusader and the diagnosticians' race with Shibasaburo Kitasoso, head of a well-funded Japanese team.[5] Again, politics raised it's not-so-pretty head as the Medical Director for the British Colony of Hong Kong hoped to tie his aspirations to the well-known Japanese Epidemeologist. Once Yersin had made his discovery, he even developed a serum by injecting horses with the bacteria (the horses survived), then using their blood to inoculate people.

This news had reached our west coast, and the physicians knew. However, the city fathers wanted no part of this truth. San Francisco was the center of culture and finance in the west, and bad news would inhibit or at least slow growth. It took many years and countless deaths before the people in authority would admit, "**It's here.**" The US Surgeon General even got pulled into the political intrigue. The first female plague death in California is well documented.

One writer described it this way: "Yellow sulfur fumes cast an amber pall over Chinatown. The Chinese choked and cursed the caustic fog. But the Health Department insisted the haze was a sign of progress against the plague. Lim Fa Muey, a teenage cigar maker, was one of those who hurried to work through the veil of chemicals one morning in early May 1900. Once she was inside the cigar factory, the familiar tang of cured tobacco leaves would have been welcome after the stench of fumigation–if she hadn't begun to feel so ill. The same symptoms that hit her neighbors now assailed the girl. They were the symptoms of a disease which officially didn't exist: the leaden ache that dragged at her back and limbs, the lurching stomach, the giddy head, the eyes that burned fever-bright. Back at her apartment at 739 Clay Street that evening, her body ached like an old woman's. Inside, the bacteria overflowed from her lymph glands into her bloodstream, invading tissues of her heart, liver and spleen. The germs' poison dissolved vessel walls, so that the blood seeped out in small hemorrhages that bloomed like ink stains beneath the skin. As her cells lost the battle against the invader, the rising fever burned her senseless. From delirium, she lapsed into coma. Her pulse sped, her organs failed. Her heart stopped. On May 11, Lin Fa Muey became San Francisco's first female plague victim, but not the last."[6] More followed until the 1950's when plague was declared managed. But around 25 million souls stepped over to the other side from this pandemic.

Few know even now, that "bubonic" is named for the buboes, which are symptomatic of the disease. They appear at sites of the lymph nodes. I still have my scar. I cannot understand why the world-class infectious disease team treating me didn't know what it was. Maybe they did, but no one was talking, again.

Much has been written on my nemesis; there are even eyewitness accounts from the not so well known first outbreak in Constantinople. One Eastern Roman Scholar, Procopius, describes vividly in his *History of the Wars* the human suffering and societal disintegration he witnessed in plague-ravaged Constantinople.[7] At the time, no one knew the origin, but everyone felt the consequences.

Fleeing was the recommended intervention. Researchers have traced the source (and continued existence of the bacteria) to central Asia, or the Steppes. The topography is desert, not unlike New Mexico's. Apparently the death-highway to the east was the Silk Road, where coveted eastern treasures made their way to a burgeoning merchant middle class of traders around Pelusium, east of Alexandria, Egypt. This was a shipping center for the region, and distribution point for the bacteria. Grain from the Nile delta was valued around the Mediterranean as a major food source, especially for bread. Varmints eat grain (they need the vitamin E). Fleas live on rats. The rats (and fleas) hitched a ride on ships carrying grain around the known world.

Rulers had no idea what to do. Emperor Justinian, a conquering warrior, had united smaller territories and politicked his way to leadership. Constantinople (currently Istanbul), was the seat of his throne. Excellent historical accounts have survived which document all manner of power seeking/ financial intrigues of the times. Commercial life was exploding, and medicine was trying to find its way, using the scientific method available in that era. However, the Catholic Church's fears that its dogmas might be undermined created suspicions which controlled experimentation and progress. Like an undernourished child, progress failed to thrive. Disease was way ahead. Anyone who lived past 40 was on borrowed time.

Meanwhile, plague was indirectly bringing major social change. That pestilence of the 3rd through the 8th centuries altered demographics, destroyed armies (who also transported plague), opened the geographic door for Mohammed's teachings (Islam), and the population move helped birth Europe. Also, a new medical intervention entered the scene: quarantine.

5. Marriott, E. Extensive story of professional rivalry. Finally 60 years after the discovery Yersin final got credit. The bacteria is called *Yersinia pestis.*

6. Chase, M. Engaging story of Plague's arrival in the USA and politics that inhibited its immediate treatment.

7. Rosen, W. Justinian's Flea. Discussion of Procopius History of the Wars.

THE SECOND PANDEMIC

There's only one thing to be said about the bubonic plague—avoid it at all costs! That's what the merchant/middle class did in the mid-14th century if they could: They ran! The members of the working class, sadly, could not. Several things kept them in the path of the tidal wave of death: They had no money for travel, they had to work at whatever occupations they had in order to survive, and were tied to their families and the community. There was not nearly the network of communication we have today, and few knew about the plague until people in their communities started dying with more frequency than usual. There were no hospitals to treat the victims, and no method to track what was happening.

People died by the millions. In most European towns it got to the point that there were more dead bodies than people to bury them. Mass graves became the answer. Some markers of those still remain. In 1997 when I was in England, a friend was driving me around London. We came upon a large open field in the midst of a combined residential and business area. I asked what that was. He told me it was the site of a mass grave from the Black Death and everyone knew what it was and respected it, though there were no headstones. I raised my eyebrows, and was quiet as I naturally showed a moment of respect. Little did I know that I could have joined them.

The death route that the plague took in the 1300's is well marked. (Researchers have even calculated the number of deaths per kilometer traveled.) Records exist from village land transfers and Bills of Mortality. [8] It made its way from China's northeastern Province of Hopei in 1334 A.D. via marmots (rodents) in Western Russia (far eastern Europe) to the Port of Caffa on the Black Sea. It probably hitched a ride along the Silk Road in caravans. Fleas, which are about the size of an ink dot from a ballpoint pin, were known to take up temporary residence in bolts of cloth, rugs and clothing being shipped from the Far East–treasures, at the time, that were being transported to the prosperous middle class. *Pulex irritans*, the human flea, has also been proposed as a carrier of the deadly bacillus.

Rodents of many species were common, but Rattus-rattus, the black one, is known to have migrated around the Mediterranean in the ancient world. It is thought to have been the primary carrier, but that was not determined until the late 19th century. Strangely, bubonic plague is chiefly a disease among rodents. Humans became convenient hosts when there were no more warm-blooded four-legged victims available. They can jump 100 times their size, which is about a meter, so they can easily jump on a human body if one is around.

Travel facilitated plague movement, and wars took the fleas onboard rats to many countries. The Hundred Years War between France and England began in 1337, and the plague went along for the ride. There is a story about an army infected with plague. It assaulted its enemy inside of walls by launching their dead into the city on catapults.[9]

Doctors at that time had no understanding of the role of bacteria in disease—or even of the existence of bacteria. Their method of treatment was to adjust the humors of the body, which were blood, yellow bile, black bile, and phlegm. Their theory was that all diseases and disabilities were the result of an excess or deficit of one of these four humors. Imbalances of the humors were thought to be caused by vapors ("bad air") inhaled or absorbed by the body. Doctors adjusted the humors through bleeding, purging, sweating and vomiting.

At the time no one knew its origin, how it was transmitted or how to cure it. Someone had to be at fault, so some blame was given to the Jews. They had more money, lived cleaner, with less incidence of plague-caused death. They also held debts, and killing them cancelled many bills.

Astrologers blamed the heavens. According to a report sent to the King of France by the medical faculty in Paris, the "great pestilence" was caused by the conjunction of three planets in 1345.

The Catholic Church was powerful, so officially, it was only "sinners" who were struck down, and only prayer and donations could possibly save the faithful. Of course they didn't.

Mostly physicians had no consistent diagnosis, and since there was no such thing as an autopsy, who really knew? A crude microscope was invented in 1590, but that did little to advance the understanding of plague. In 1665 Dr. Nathaniel Hodges published a description of a case he had diagnosed: "Two risings about the bigness of a nutmeg broke out, one on each thigh; upon examination of which I soon discovered the malignancy, both from their black hue and the circle around them; and pronounced it to be plague, in which opinion I was subsequently confirmed."[10] This was 300 years after the 1350 outbreak.

A cross was painted on homes of plague victims, which is how the symbol for the Red Cross organization originated. Those afflicted were grouped together in plague houses (quarantine).

However, the plague was not the only lethal agent at the time. A weakened immune system was also prey to typhoid fever, tuberculosis, syphilis, smallpox, yellow fever, influenza, cholera, meningitis, staphylococcal toxic shock, heart attacks, high blood pressure, anthrax, ebola, polio, chickenpox, and hanta virus. Only the plague had buboes as a symptom.

The rampage did not suddenly stop. It continued: Venice in 1624 reported 142,804 deaths, then 98,244 in1633. Pope Clement estimated 23,840,000 died out of a population of 75 million. One book characterized London's worst year of deaths as 1665 when 68,956 known deaths occurred.[11]

8. Slack, P. Excellent demographics in a brief work

9. Cantor, N. In The Wake of the Plague

10. Moote, L. and Moote, D.

11. Ibid.

STILL IN THE HOSPITAL

About the third or fourth day of my life-changing odyssey, I briefly came out of my stupor. Through one eye I saw the medical staff wearing surgical masks, which they hadn't done before. Visitors that day wore them, too. Nobody seemed to really know what I had—at least they weren't telling me! I wasn't that surprised. I found out later that the concern was that I might contaminate others with my mysterious condition by coughing. My lungs were filling with fluid; pneumonia loomed.

There is one form of the plague, pneumonic, that is airborne, and kills within a day or two. Remember the nursery rhyme: "Ring around the rosy (darkness surrounding the bubo), pocket full of posey (pus/poison). Achoo!. Achoo! We all fall down!" That is attributed to the pneumonic form, which is communicated through the air and makes straight for the lungs.

It was only after a blood culture test conducted by state laboratories that the diagnosis was confirmed. Plague takes 10 days to incubate and be positively identified through tests. Thankfully the doctors had started treating me with antibiotics immediately. The antibiotics were developed during World War II; prior to that, there was no known cure. Until the diagnosis was made, no one could (or would) tell me much of anything about my situation. I kept losing weight, receiving sustenance and medications through tubes, lying helplessly except when the physical therapists came to roust me to make me walk.

The memory of their first attempt is so clear to me. With hardly any physical strength, it took all I had to sit up in bed. Then I tried to cover my butt, which is impossible in a hospital gown. Someone put a walker in front of me and coaxed me to stand. I didn't like it. They had to help me up. I almost fell over. After a few shuffling steps I said to myself, "I'll never walk again." Only a week before I had been out in the woods cutting trees, physically active at almost age 60. Never did I imagine I'd be here, trying to walk, questioning life again.

On subsequent days when the physical therapists appeared, I grimaced. Not only was I weak, my body temperature fluctuated wildly. At various times I'd perspire, then shake due to chills probably in part due to all of the drugs I was receiving. This often happened on walks (or corridor shuffles). Once I was about 30 steps down the hallway and began shaking, almost to convulsion. Someone threw a thin hospital blanket around me, and cheered me on to amble back to bed...GRRRR. They were merciless and persistent. But their coaching over the six weeks was useful. I had a shoulder pain that they helped me with also. I guess that I had fallen before admission, perhaps when I blacked out at home. It still isn't completely healed.

The major symptom of the plague is infection. That's how it kills us. The deadly bacillus masks itself–actually evades detection by our immune systems. Usually pneumonia is the cause of death. Many plague-related deaths go unreported, because plague has disguised itself. Lungs fill with fluid: no air, no life.

Upon my arrival in the ICU, I received oxygen through two little dispensers in my nose. Since I was mostly unconscious for the first two weeks, I did not notice my labored breathing, but the ICU staff did. A friendly young volunteer appeared one day, saying that I was going to see the lung specialist. They, again, got no resistance from me. An affable lady doctor described the procedure for removing fluid. I was surprised; still am. She showed me an implement that looked like a yard rake, except it had a short handle with short steel tines about three to four inches long. Now this could all be delusion, but it seemed real to me. I bent over a table, after signing the usual release, and she ran the rake up and down my back. After about thirty minutes she showed me a container that looked like a liter of soda; except that it contained material sucked out of my lungs, through my skin. The things they can do are amazing. I learned so much about science and medical technology through this "catastrophe." Too bad I had to do it the hard way.

PLAGUE SPEAKS (FINALLY)

The Steppes are a desert-like, almost barren area stretching from Ukraine in the west through Russia, Kazakhstan, Turkmenistan and Uzbekistan. Plague had to start somewhere, and it's believed it was in the Steppes. Scientists suggest that Ms. Nature evolved the plague bacteria to manage the varmint population in that region (if we even consider that "she" thinks about things like this). Russia still has a standing committee on plague management. The threat of plague is just one more-harsh factor associated with living in the former Soviet Union.

One day I was musing and asked myself what plague would say if it could speak. This is the dialogue that came to me.

(Michael) M: *What in the hell is this all about? You wiped out so many of us, and now I learn it was never intended to affect humans? Come on!*

(Plague) P: *Don't blame me. Not my fault. He/ She or It did it.*

M: *Who's this she? I don't care: He, She, It or some god somewhere. I don't like this suffering I've been through.*

P: *But isn't that the truth: Poor you just doesn't like the way things are— life is on life's terms, pal. Your complaining is more of life on Michael's terms. More knowledge isn't going to give you more control. The truth is that you all just got in "my way."*

M: *It's a human thing to escape my own responsibility in my own life, I guess. I can still ask the same question asked of me: 'Why didn't someone tell me New Mexico is the land of the flea and home of the plague?' Half of the cases a year in the USA are here, and no one knows it!*

P: *You think the good city or state fathers want to advertise that? Part of my success is that when I show up, people go into denial. That helps my progress, a lot. Always has.*

P: Take your choice. I'm busy evolving so I can keep going. I understand researchers keep track of me, yet there isn't much going on in the antibiotic department. You guys just react when I come up with something new. A few years ago there was that strain which none of your drugs could kill. I'm one up on you.

HERE'S THE MESSAGE:

BE CAREFUL. BUBONIC PLAGUE IS ALIVE AND WELL,

PERHAPS IN YOUR NEIGHBORHOOD!

SHADOW RETURNS

My previous conversation left me with more questions than answers: I was lying in my own emotional and psychological vomit. I reeked of *"Ok, I'm alive, but just barely; now what? Why did I survive when millions didn't? What's my purpose now? How am I going to find it? Damn, I can barely move, so how is this purpose going to find me?"* Just as my head was trying to find a way out of this, Keith showed up. He'd always been able to help me make sense of confusion. He listened quietly. Calmly he said, "Maybe you ought to get well first. I recommend you walk, and worry later; and prayer wouldn't hurt either." He was right, as usual. Days earlier he had the same effect on me when I was concerned about paying the medical bill.

Usually when I calmed, I slept. Anyone with hospital experience knows that napping is the replacement for solid hours of sleep. Noise and interruption inhibit rest–so then, rest, Michael. As he sat there at peace, I dozed. With no difficulty I found myself re-engaged in a conversation with Muerto. No introductions were necessary. From the tone and arrogance I knew it was he.

Death (D): You're still fussing. Trying to understand, aren't you? You never will!

Michael (M): I'm seeing that I've just got to accept absolutely. It's that way for me–I bloody my head by banging it against something long enough to realize I've got to quit; then I stop bleeding and see that's what's needed all along. And you, Mr. Death, are just another fact of this life for me to accept. You know that there have been several times that I've been aware of your presence. I remember a few years ago when I told a friend you were near. Getting my affairs in order, I prepared to go. But no invitation to cross over was forthcoming. What happened?

D: That one I remember. You may not think it, but this hospital time has been good for you. Your brush with me is getting you more ready. I am not your enemy. People fear me. I am the natural part of life–just the next step.

M: I'm getting that, slowly; but you are not my friend, yet, either. But perhaps could you be? Or as you said, the next step after a flower blooms is the dried-up blooms. Roses don't last forever, either. As a kid I remember building an elaborate city in the sand box out back which my father had made. Next day when I went out the cats had used city hall and my roadway as their litter box. So much for things lasting. So now, as a big boy I get to face that things (even me) don't last forever. I wonder what's next ? Could there be freedom in this disattachment? My friend the monk talks about being ready 'to go' in each breath, not waiting:

For something else to make me happy

To thank someone, or tell the truth, now

To spend an extra moment, savoring...whatever

To linger to embrace the 'eye-lock' with a stranger

To part from a loved one as if it might be the last time I'll see them, hear their voice, or touch their skin

To dawdle a moment to really enjoy whatever that moment provides.

Then go to the next breath, perhaps in a new place with (or without) another.

D: If you could only disconnect from 'that mind' that runs you, Michael. You can't know it all, anyway. Ha, it's not even your mind. Let go! Enjoy the trip. Everything works out, one way or the other, with or without your hands on it. The sea comes in and the sea goes out. Surf the wave of life. Ski the mountain until spring. Follow the sunshine if you'd like. Or keep suffering because things don't go your way. That's what you've been doing, you know. Your depression? It's been you demanding that life go your way, then getting discouraged because it can't all of the time. Too simple? Try it on. And tell the truth.

M: I do not like this. But it's pretty close to 'right-on'. And it makes sense to me, though I never realized I was suffering just because I didn't get what I wanted. How underhanded and self-punishing. I've seen others get what they want, why can't I?

D: You think you're alone in this question? People want what they want when they want it—and they figure out how to get it; then they suffer because that's not enough, either. You all take, take, take. Until at some point you wake up to your own craziness. "He who dies with the most toys wins" Right? Isn't that the American way? Wins what? You all ain't gonna beat me.

M: You're right about that. But I've never been into 'toys'—experiences, yes. In my family we weren't big on possessions—we never had much, except each other. From an early age I learned how to take care of others. Getting the things I wanted seemed to come after others getting theirs. I really always wanted more, though.

D: Michael, life happens life's way. You never learned that—to live with life on life's terms. For you, acceptance is going to be the key to your happiness; and doing what you can for others. The lessons you got in your family were the right ones. Your job from now on is to help others. What's left of your life is not about you, anymore—that is, if you want to live the rest of it happy, joyous and free. I've watched you since you were a child...good kid in a good family, good education that you worked for. But there was a latent rebel in you. For years you lived by others rules, questioning, until you had a chance to try the "other side." That didn't make you happy, either, did it? What's it going to take for you to get it? You don't have much time left—there's a lot more behind you than ahead. Has your attention been gotten yet? Wake up!

M: All right! So, that's it, eh; that simple? Help others and take myself out of the equation?

D: You will get as you give. Haven't you always been taken care of? Stop the complicating. and keep being open.

M: I can try—but I see how selfish and self-centered I am. Not living in fear, helping others freely, expecting nothing in return—that's a major change for me. Even liking it?

D: You can do this, I know. By the way, do you know what an angel is?

M: What's this angel stuff? Sure, they watch over us, and do miracles, I'm told.

D: Yes and no. It's not mystical. Your parents were angels; they didn't know it, though. Didn't they watch over you and try to guide you, as well as carry Her message to you? Here's the news—you have it in you, too. Helping *others was their job and yours too. There's no mystery to it. Remember that guy named Angel when you were six years sober and that time over coffee? He told you that he had a message for you; then what he said?*

M: *Sure, he looked at me very intently, and told me a story about when he was a trucker with a CB handle of "Kentucky Blue Bird." Once a song came on the radio that got his attention. It was something like: "Fly away, Kentucky Blue Bird, and take a message to Michael...." So he got in his truck, drove to Louisville, walked into a meeting, saw a guy with an "M" on his belt buckle who was holding a guitar. (The other part to the song is "Take a message to Michael, he's playing in some café..."). Angel walked up to him and asked if his name was Michael, and if he was playing in a café. The fellow said, "Yes." Angel then looked at me, after he had captivated me with this story, and said, "I have a message for you!"*

"OK", I said with anticipation, "What is it?"

Quietly, he leaned forward, as if it were a secret, and whispered to me, "I will always love you, so." Tears came to my eyes as I let that in. It was as if the Laser Light of the Universe got through to my soul. I could say nothing. He sat back and chuckled, like he had gotten one over on me—which he had. That moment still touches me, right now. Over the years I've repeated that story to a few others, when conditions were just right. Only when they seemed ready did I do it, as it's a pretty personal and special moment.

D: *Absolutely. But everyone needs it. Carry that message! You are working on your wings. All of you can be angels, not always to everyone all of the time; but human beings can do it. They just don't know it. Mostly, people don't own it. The idea seems too arrogant to them. After all, they say, "Could I really be an angel?" That would mean that you'd have to live up to it by living honorably, wouldn't it? See? My message to you: "You are loved, now get after it!" I'm waiting for you....*

ENOUGH OF ICU

As I began to feel somewhat human, I got the word that I was to be moved from the ICU to a smaller, less modern hospital room. My mementos had to go too. I had accumulated almost a garbage bag full of minutiae given to me by friends while I was under 24/7 care: cards, a plant or two, magazines from guys (either about cars or guns), and books. All of that was extra luggage I really didn't want any longer. The presence of the people who had given them is what had helped; and what I had needed—not the material things they gave me. I was getting ready for a different place. How soon would I go?

Big Nurse delivered the news. Waddling into the room pronouncing: "You'll live and we need this room—you're getting moved!" Just like that, matter of fact. What happened to the comforting bedside manner? By being with these medical folks for a while, I'd discovered something: they are human, too, in all of the variety of sizes, personality types and expressions of compassion. Some took their profession as a calling under a mission to serve. Others, like this Nurse Ratchet, were burned out, collecting a paycheck, and "just doin' their eight until they hit the gate." Mostly it didn't matter much. I didn't take it personally.

"When?" I queried.

"When there's a room," she snapped. From her tone I caught her unspoken word, "Dummy."

Then that mind started in on me, worrying and fussing. I told myself, "*Just sit tight, pal. You've had your first shave in two weeks by a good friend. But it's September, so this summer is gone, and you need to get ready for cold weather. What about your house in the mountains? Where will you get firewood for the winter? Who's going to put tar around those pesky skylights that occasionally leak? How about the heat tape on those water pipes? Think they'll hold for another winter? Is the chimney clean enough? And that old truck with 300,000 miles. It may not make it through the winter."* On and on, I'd been listening to it for 60 years. Did you ever tell "It" to shut up, then notice what happens next? "It" starts up, again. <u>That mind has a mind of its own</u>, to quote one of my favorite bumper stickers. More often than not I (whatever that is) am so in the "chatter" before I recognize that I'm listening (or who is speaking). "The Voice," I've heard it labeled; or called "monkey mind". Whatever the name, that entity is true for all of us—and has us do very crazy things.

Thirty-five years ago someone pointed <u>It</u> out to me saying, "Sit quietly, close your eyes and *listen!*" It responded, "What chatter? He's crazy, there's no voice speaking." Then, bingo, I heard <u>It</u> for the first time. Now <u>It</u> had gone off once more, and I (whatever this is) was <u>Its</u> prisoner. My zen monk friend, not too kindly, beat me over the head about this, regularly. Actually I call him a Rude-ist monk as he works in a prison. He says that he is ruthlessly compassionate. No matter. It is alive and still screaming at me. And the "I", the self, is a mystery or work-in-progress.

Without much fanfare, my body and goods got moved to the smaller room, in hospital time. Three weeks of intense 24/7 scrutiny gave way to a more compact space, by myself in an older wing of the main hospital. At least there was a window for contact with the outside world, even if it did look out at a brick wall...air and sunshine, at last. After two weeks of stabilization there I was to be moved again. The next available bed was at a longer-term rehabilitation unit. I was getting better. Finally, the medical world was letting me in on my recovery.

Apparently the wound-vacuum attached to my arm was not a unit with which one was released. Changing the sponge pad on the wound to which the suction was attached was a very big deal. The procedure took every pain-killing drug that I was prescribed, plus four orderlies holding me down—men who could play linebacker for a professional football team. Add in one compassionate nurse-all to remove a 4 by 6-inch compress off of my arm. The problem was that there happened to be new growth of skin attached to it. My God, did that hurt! It made me understand more about the techniques of torture.

An hour or so before the procedure every other morning, a nurse would bring in and hang a drip bag of morphine, which was intended to deaden the pain. How can anyone think that anything, short of being unconscious, could stop the agony of peeling a covering off of a wound that is attached to a fresh layer of skin? Besides, narcotics usually do not have a pain-deadening effect on me—I get high, then crazy. That is, I get fearful, regrets from the past resurface, and shame. Medical morphine did not make me crave more; but I did like the intoxicating feeling I got. One time a nurse gave me a Percoset then a dose of morphine. It did not anesthetize me. My system was probably getting used to processing it. I reported this to her. She came back with another syringe and shot it into a previously placed receiver in my arm. OHHH, YEAHHH! That got it, Nursey! Wow, a peace and relaxation came over me that I hadn't felt in years. A calm, like all tension melting and "that mind" switched off in favor of a body that had let go of any stress. I didn't feel anything. And everything around me was just fine the way it was, however it was, over and out! I'm sure I slurred my words as I tried to speak. But in spite of my relaxation, the gauze change was excruciating.

Right there, at that point was when my recovery support became most clear. Immediately following the procedure I felt a huge relief that it was over. Then the fears and tears would begin. One of the members of my support team of friends suggested that they plan their visits to coincide with the completion of the compress changing. Brilliant! During the next post-pain process, I clearly remember saying through my tears, " I don't want to go back (to addiction)." And someone said, "We won't let you." They didn't.

Aside from this, that phase was also memorable for the afternoon nurse on duty, Kathleen. Her appearance let me know that I was still among the living. In her late thirties, had a half-dozen facial piercings and a streak of purple running down the middle of her short red hair, worn twice as long on the right side as the left. More than her striking appearance, it was the air of pain about her that caught my attention. She went about her nursing tasks deliberately, in a low-key manner, saying little until I asked, "How are you?"

She snapped her head 90 degrees to the left, looked directly at me, and said, "I've had better days." I liked her spontaneity and the fact that she gave me an honest answer instead of indicating that everything was fine.

"What do you mean?" I asked.

She took a couple of steps toward me, put her right hand on her hip and shot back "I have two young boys I'm raising alone. Their father was killed last year."

I gulped silently and responded, "That does make life tough, doesn't it?"

"Yes, and my mother-in-law baby-sits my boys and sometimes pisses me off, like this morning." An attitude came at me along with the words.

After a quiet moment's reflection, I responded "There is a price to pay for everything, even free babysitting. She probably wants to help, just doesn't know how."

"Yes, but I'm the mom and she tries to take over a lot, then the boys get confused when she tells them things opposite from my rules!"

Wanting to be understanding, but also help her into a solution, I said, "That seems to be how it is, raising kids; and being a single mom with boys is even tougher. Can you talk to her about this?"

"Yes, but I miss him. We used to talk about stuff. He was a really good man and father—we all miss him so." Her tone lightened a bit. What could anyone say to that?

"Grandma is not a replacement, that's for sure. But if you could talk to her about this I bet you'd feel better." I said. "I'm sure you're a good mom, and they know it. You know, I'm trapped in this room for a while, and I'll trade you some listening for nursing service. How's that?"

Smiling now, she said, "I'll do that, anyway, but thanks. I needed to blow off some steam. What's your name? What are you here for?" And I told her the story from the beginning.

KASEMAN TIME

The last leg of the hospital journey was by no means the least adventuresome. When the EMT's came to the main hospital to transport me to the Kaseman long-term recovery facility, they rightfully spent more time securing my body to the gurney than packing my earthly belongings into a garbage bag. Then they called for an ambulance. Doing their job, the EMT's were on task, but engaged me in conversation. As I was tightly tucked in, exiting the room, tears came to my eyes. Something life altering had happened there and I was about to leave. Goodbyes have never been easy for me, especially when I was about to pass from a place where I was snatched from Señor Muerto. One attendant noticed my teary eyes and asked, "Are the straps too tight?"

"No" I said. "Just saying goodbye and thank you to the room." His head nodded to the right, then left, as he looked like he was processing a mystery. I've seen that very same response elsewhere; for instance, in my dog when she doesn't understand. But at least the medical transport guy could say, "Oh." Ms. Dog just wonders what in the hell I'm doing. He let it slide also. With me packed tightly on my bundling board-on-wheels, accompanied by a huge garbage bag containing three weeks' worth of paraphernalia, we headed for the ambulance; but not before I nodded a "thank you" to the staff at the 6th floor desk. That small gesture of appreciation did not convey the full measure of gratitude I felt at that moment. At the desk the middle-aged nurse, Nancy, who had held my hand during skin-removal, answered my frantic middle-of-the-night calls for help, and changed my soaking-wet gown more than once as I detoxed, simply smiled as I passed. I'm not a lip-reader, but it wasn't hard to discern her variation of "You're welcome." Off we went to the next adventure.

After a short but probably expensive ride, we arrived at the new facility. As I rolled into a new room, a welcoming attendant, perhaps a nurse, smiled me in. He appeared Arabic, and soon I saw his name was Mohammed. Almost instinctively, I said, "As salamu alaykum." His head jerked back an inch or two in surprise. "Wa Alaicum Salaam," he responded. As I was taught in Riyadh, that is the spiritual greeting in the Muslim world. Once again I knew I was in good hands, watched over by the Spirit of the Universe, by whatever Name it goes by.

Taken care of by a Higher Power is one thing, but foremost in my mind was, *"When do I go home?"* Nobody seemed to know, nor did there seem to be anyone who could or would address my query. I was beginning to doubt that I would ever be discharged, and probably some of the staff were thinking the same thing. As progressive as medicine has become in the last seventy years, almost any physician (when honest, with no witnesses present) will tell you that their profession is a well-informed crapshoot with loaded dice. Based on prior experience (along with documentation of medical school cases) they take their best shot at healing. Drugs come with warning labels about lethal doses, but plague's healing processes are at best a play-it-by-ear set of protocols. There was no road map. Clearly I was stabilized. However, the longer one stays in that environment, the better the chances become of an infection from some renegade bug. Between the high-dollar wound vacuum attached to my arm and my wobbly walking, it didn't look like I was headed for home anytime soon. As fretting set in, so did a memory of a time when I was employed at a treatment center for adolescents. When it was time for discharge, a plan was created–by the social worker. There had to be such a person in this place. When the charge nurse made her next shift-change rounds, I popped the magic question, "Is there a discharge planner here?"

"Of course" was her assertive response. "She's right down the hall, two doors past the nurses' station."

Soon thereafter I hobbled my way down to that office. Upon the first attempt no one was home. A couple of hours later I tried again, and this time a harried-looking thirtyish lady opened that door, and I judged from her appearance that she had to be the person. It was that hospital social worker look: a bit overweight, frumpy to the max, cluttered desk with a no doubt equally messy mind, overworked, way behind on her paperwork. Yep, this was not going to go smoothly. When I gave her the Cliff Notes of my situation, she wrote down my name and room number. I could always count on "I'm in here recovering from the bubonic plague" to get someone's attention. It had this time, I hoped.

But frankly, I just wanted out of there; almost enough to go AMA—"against medical advice": abscond, boogie, take off, head back home. Not that my private room was some kind of dungeon. With TV, phone, hot-and-cold running volunteers wanting to meet the "plague boy," I wasn't suffering in the creature comfort department. But patience never has been my long suit, so I punctuated my days with distractions. They usually started before dawn with the cable channel that featured a station playing classical music, beautiful sequences of landscapes with quotations from the Bible. In a pinch (which this was) those scripture verses, especially the Psalms (David's songs of praise to Yahweh) settled that feisty early morning mind. About the time I couldn't take any more of that, the workers started arriving at the construction site across the street. That large piece of glass on the north side of my room was a window to the world.

Almost like on a big-screen TV, I got to watch the Construction Channel playing over there. Exterior metal framing of a soon-to-be-doctors' office was in place with interior walls being erected. That was clear because windows were in place as the workmen were siding her, with the sheetrock truck using the boom to place drywall onto the second floor. (Man, did I ever love that work as a carpenter, then foreman, ultimately becoming a superintendent on a job at Los Alamos National Laboratory.) I took daily attendance, noted who was violating safety standards, what was not being done according to the code, with or without correction. This took a good hour in the morning. Vital signs, breakfast, medications, some physical therapy (mostly relearning to walk) took me till about noon. In between were opportunities for naps, crossword puzzles, specialists who consulted sporadically, but not one of them with a "kick out" date or criteria for it. This was a high level limbo. Faithful friends' visits became less frequent, since they knew I was going to live through this one. A few days after my arrival, though, it felt like the military had landed.

The Veterans

Four male friends came laughing their way into my DMZ chamber. First was the trim squad leader, Randy, the point man. He was a quiet volcano, one whose eruption no one would want to experience. He had around TEN lock ups under his belt, and none of us knew how many were jails and how many were mental hospitals. He couldn't remember either, probably as a result of one too many ECT's (Electro-Convulsive Therapies—shock treatments). It all started in Nam.

Next marched in Ranger Jim, the Army sniper. As a poker-faced, stocky fellow, he was not unlike a small tank. He invented covert operations, for one minute he was here, the next he was gone. Believe me, this is one well-trained fellow whom you'd not want to piss off. There was good reason to have him as a friend since he had no fear of any human being.

Then Williams wandered in behind the first two. This guy played his cards very close to his vest, never really saying what he did in the Army. We all knew he was brilliant, likely an analyst of some sort, given his short stature and shifty eyes. Once he let slip some Chinese when one of the team told a joke about Ho Chi Min.

Covering the rear was Motorcycle Michael, a longhaired street vet still clawing his way out of the Southeast Asian jungle. His eyes were continually surveying the environment–hyper-vigilance it's called. But you could sure count on him to keep the rear end covered. Nothing was going to get by him, alive. If one took time to consider the idea, this country is quite safe from invasion: all of the weapons, all of the vets, all of the leftover paranoia are still here–maybe they're just looking for a reason to go back "out there."

Having them together in that place really, really made my day. Of course, each in turn had to comment or ask a question to which the others responded with a jocular remark. *"Now you did it, son,"* spoke the elder Randy, though younger than I. Like the typical southern sheriff who would say "Boy," he said "Son." That's just the way he is. There was concern in his eyes and tone, but indirectly, as he's not one to express feelings overtly.

Guys are like that–sometimes the message is hidden between the lines. Though I am one of them (men), being raised mostly under my mom's influence, it has taken me a long time to adjust into that male thing. My first realization of this disparity came in college when I did the Minnesota Multiphasic Personality Inventory (commonly known as MMPI), ultimately being told by the counselor that I scored high on the female index. That horrified me. Was I gay? No, just answered questions like a woman would... Ruth's tutelage. That's probably why I liked construction–the guy thing was pretty strong in the trades; and I could banter with the best of them. Not being athletic, a rugged kind of maleness in my youth did not fit me. Mandatory locker room antics in high school were uncomfortable at best and embarrassing at worst.

Talking "smack," that one-up thing we do, happens almost all of the time whenever two or more "testeron-ics" are gathered. Mostly it's verbal judo. My family of origin was all about that–who could outdo the other in Jedi, Light Saber dueling, using words, tone of voice, facial expressions. Survival was based on achieving the upper hand, or at least not being one down. After years of training at stiletto-type, close-hand verbal competition, I developed a quick wit. Manipulating dialogue using a kind of blaming humor became second nature. In the real world, assessing the other when engaging a stranger is essential. That's just human. But searching out weak spots, the soft underbelly where each of us is vulnerable to that painful slight or criticism–that was my forte. I even invented a word, "sarfecious," which combined sarcastic and facetious as an art form. Even lying in that bed, incapacitated, that mind was well connected to this mouth. What went through one, often, automatically came out the other. But dealing with men requires a set of skills more related to safety. A wrong word perceived as too much threat could result in a physical counterattack. At the home training camp we were mostly safe from bodily retribution, except when the victim ran to Mom with tears in the equation.

As the oldest of seven, it seemed there was a level of responsibility (or culpability) that befell me. "Parentized" is the term for being co-opted into a junior parent role, which is what happened to me. My two younger brothers, Tim and Dan, were more in the menace category, certainly not a threat. In the old neighborhood I had two good pals: Robert and Jerry. Their older brothers were bullies who taught me lessons in careful selection of words. Later, high school in the big city brought a whole new crowd of guys to deal with. That's where I really learned the art of mouth management. It's no doubt that this is where I accepted part of the myth of manhood.

In the turbulent decade of the 60's it seemed that everyone began to question everything, much to the chagrin of institutions and inquirers alike. The unpopular war in Vietnam fueled ideas, even questions about what constituted manhood. Is/was it right to step into others' lives to help, whether they wanted assistance or not? Force? What kind and how much is appropriate? Where does "flower power" fit in: Peace, Love, Expanding Consciousness? There were always more questions than answers, and those questions led me to seek medicine for my troubled soul in the form of alcohol and drugs. Though I thought I was alone, I wasn't. A whole generation of us was groping our way through the cultural darkness.

Then, that day into my recovery room marched four of my close male friends, my age, all military veterans who had tried to "make things right." Fully trained in the art of war, scarred by the same, wiser for the lessons, they had survived. One of them, the sniper/assassin, had talked to me very personally a year before. Having had some training in martial arts, I reflected that I could kill if I had to. His response: "It's not a big deal to take another's life, war gives you permission. Living with it afterwards, that's the test. I've drawn blood, taken shrapnel, carried a dead brother out of a firefight then left it all over there. My dad did that when he came back from Europe. When he took off his uniform, then that was that. Of course he ended up drinking those memories away. Me? I'm here in the Albuquerque "war zone" neighborhood teaching boys in shop class."

He drew close to me as I lay there in my own MASH unit bed, bent down and whispered, "You need anything, anytime you call. I'll be here." That's count-on-ability. Ultimate trust is built on the firing line...you live or die together.

The warrior tradition goes back a long ways, and not just in myth: Samurai awakened to: "It's a good day to die," then went out to serve. There's something in that kind of experience that I haven't had in this lifetime, but in the previous one I did. What do I mean by that? All of us baby boomers were in an earlier war. I believe strongly that we returned here to complete unfinished lessons interrupted by our premature deaths in World War II.

No matter, these guys survived. These friends were wounded healers. Not only had each fought the enemy outside, but their own demons. I respected them absolutely. Having been to hell, they decided to have no more of the self-inflicted pain of over-or under-the-counter medicine. Done with the soul imprinted with anguish, their new mission is to assist others so afflicted. That is honor in action.

They can sometimes speak of the softer side: feelings, compassion and tenderness. They can write poetry, create art, and be kind. Though able to be a bit softer, their underlying roughness can still be resurrected when needed. Into this rehab facility they brought me a direct lesson that I did not really want to hear. Randy, not so politely said, "When are you going to get your ass out of that bed, son?"

Everything in me wanted to shoot back some kind of smart remark, but I knew he was asking a serious question in his own way. I squeaked out my response. "Brother, this thing has kicked my ass. Some days not only can't I move, I almost don't want to."

Obviously he didn't want to hear my excuses. "Same thing happened to me in Nam," he said. "Shrapnel laid me up for two months. You think I wanted to jump right up and head back into that jungle bullshit? Not without good drugs–hell, I got better dope on the streets of Saigon. I know what it's like to lay there with the life beat out of you. You can do that if you want, but that's not you."

"Come on," I fired back, "give me a break. I've lost 35 pounds in three weeks, have night sweats from the drugs, am still dealing with this skin-sucker on my arm, and have no idea when I'm getting out of here. Lighten up on me!"

"Poor baby," Williams said with his own sarfecious inflection, almost sing-song. A tone clearly intended to deepen the verbal wound. It did...like the twist of a knife once inserted.

"OK, what do you want from me?" I said, surrendering. All four of the squad looked at each other at once. They each seemed to know what the others were thinking. Then they went into a huddle, arms around one another. I knew something was coming. After what seemed like a long time, but probably wasn't, they lined up at the end of my bed, looked seriously at me, then said together, "Don't give up, we're here for you!"

Then the ringleader said more softly, tilting his head, raising one eyebrow a bit, "You're sunk if you don't fight for your own life. Healing takes guts. Reach down in there and find your purpose, again. You did it once when you kicked dope. Sorry, that's the truth."

At that I relaxed. "You're right," I said. "But I just don't have it in me for this fight. Getting out of this bed to take a shit wipes me out. Walking ten steps, I have to stop to catch my breath. I hate waking up in the night soaking wet with the shivers. Detox from so many drugs, I guess. Sometimes I can't or don't even want to call the nurse for help. I just don't wanna, anymore."

In the middle of this conversation a strange insight came to me: I had whined my way through life; and here it was, again. The easier, softer way has been complaining, grumbling about damned near everything that didn't go my way, blaming something or somebody for my poor pitiful condition. Then I remembered what my coach said when I expressed dismay at having my defects of character removed. "Michael," he said, "it's just willingness."

THE BABY

On a day when I'd finally had enough of that bed and jail-cell-like room, I gathered my gumption (and a robe) for an excursion down the hallway. Out the door, I first had to trundle past the nurses' station on the left directly across from where I called home. For some strange reason, I felt like I needed medical permission, which I didn't. Though they were in charge of almost every important aspect of my life such as meals, medication, clean bedding and smocks, visitations and contact with the outside world, they seemed glad to see me on my feet, smiling as I crept by; with a nod that almost said, "We see you. Have a nice trip." In itself, getting up and moving was an act of personal accomplishment, and for sure an exercise in balance. All I had to do to motivate myself to walk was to remember that a month earlier I could barely stand. Getting going was not out of some sense of a laudable push to heal. Rather, it was boredom combined with a need to move. Life is like that sometimes: what appears from the outside to be an act of heroism more often is driven by desperation. To leave that facility, I had to walk.

Typical for a long-term recovery unit, this place was laid out on a grid, not unlike city blocks, except intersections were 20 feet apart. Thankfully walls were stout enough to support my weight when I took a rest stop every ten steps or so. Passers-by would ask if I was all right. I'd smile and say, "Yes, just catching my breath." What I really wanted to tell them was, *"I just survived the bubonic plague, trying to walk again, full of drugs that are making me crazy, lonely, trying to keep it together—and you want to know how I'm doing?"*

A volunteer gave me a wheelchair that I pushed/leaned on, which also carried the wound vacuum attached to my left upper arm. It went everywhere I did. Not large (about shoe-box sized), nor heavy (a couple of pounds), but enough to throw off the gait of a guy relearning to walk. There are so many things taken for granted—almost unconscious—that a physical thumping brings back to the here-and-now. Hauling one's body, albeit forty pounds lighter, down a corridor was one. The plague had relieved me of a lot of physical strength along with a quarter of my body weight, probably mostly muscle. I felt like an explorer headed out on an adventure only half prepared. Most visitors were there out of kindness, willing to help, so of course I could always park myself in the rolling chair and wait for a charitable soul to push me back to shore. On that first foray I only made it around the "block," mostly offices. But halfway around I discovered a long line of ceiling-to-floor windows, with a door that opened to a courtyard enclosed on all four sides by the building. There were flowers, grass, and a rock garden with a couple of benches at the far left end. However, I was thwarted from entering by a locked door. I shrugged and headed back to the room, hearing myself say, "I'm too tired, anyway."

It was late summer, still warm enough not to have to bundle up, except my body temperature was unpredictable. Women with hot flashes had nothing on me, but mine were cold flashes with shivers that would come on unexpectedly. The wound vacuum sat on an extra blanket, just for good measure.

The next morning, after the usual medical procedures had been completed, found me anxious for another run at the corridors, maybe even the courtyard. Loading up the walking assistor, I almost couldn't wait to round that last bend and head for the wall of glass. Strangely I didn't rest quite as often, this trip, as I had on the previous day. Then, there it was! And someone was just exiting my entrance door. Like a racer headed for the finish line, I summoned what strength I had left, shot headlong ten feet, shoving the wheelchair between the door and the jamb. Whew! Now I had to rest a moment before heading out to that almost-outdoor space. I could see the other three walls were office spaces with windows to this little chunk of nirvana amid medical sterility: obviously a perk for a Vice President of something-or-other. Inching into the rolling chair, I moved myself out there. That was awkward, bumping over brick pavers, using arm muscles I hadn't employed for a while.

Gardeners must have just pulled weeds or planted bushes, for a strong, earthy scent hit me. Wow, I hadn't gotten that one for so long–there is no other smell to equal it. As they sang in Oklahoma!, "When the wind comes right behind the rain...." Then the calm became noticeable–no controlled environment, like the one I had been in for a month. Here and there, patches of sunlight hit parts of the wall and ground. And it was warm, not the constant 70-degree air-conditioned world I'd left behind. No PA announcing, "Doctor Red, stat to the ER!" Flies buzzed around. It was like a greenhouse without a roof. Coaxing my body over to a bench, I propped in the corner against the armrest, exhaled a big breath, and sat. Time stopped. Birds chatted to one another. Noisy bees were visiting flowers nearby, looking for honey makin's. Arms rested in my lap, going numb. Head went back as far as it could as I heard my measured breaths in-and-out, like I never had before. Peace settled upon me. That mind seemed to shut down for a bit—at least the volume lowered. Perhaps I dozed off, because I startled myself awake with a snort. Head snapped forward, eyes popped open, hands moved an inch or two, and I was back in this garden world. Of course I was not wearing a watch, so I had no idea what time it was, nor did I care.

After a while, perhaps twenty minutes or so, a couple disturbed the calm by entering my space, chortling to one another as they came through the door. He with a leg in a cast, on crutches, in his thirties, sporting a hospital robe. A cute gal was beside him, being attentive. They looked to need some privacy, so up I got, shuffling back in "there." Just as I re-entered the sterile environment, checking to make sure no one got T-boned with the wheelchair, I looked to the right and saw them.

She was coming down the hall with a little guy holding her left hand. He had on shorts, sneakers, a tie-dyed tee shirt, sunglasses and a baseball cap. All of about three feet tall, next to her five foot or so, he seemed happy, sporting a big smile. I stopped dead in my tracks as they came the fifteen feet toward me. Her shoulder-length brunette hair bounced against tanned shoulders that held two small straps of a yellow cotton summer dress. She was a cutie. There was a bundle around her middle, below her full breasts, but above her waist, attached around her neck with a wide strap. It was a newborn. As they came within a few steps of me I said, *"Wow, a new arrival."*

"Yep, just two months old." Not hesitating a moment, she pulled back the cover to reveal a round-faced little one with the bluest eyes, wearing a cap similar to the one worn by the young chap at her side. In the length of a breath, that baby and I locked eyes and he smiled. Philosophers discuss that moment of "beholding." In those few seconds a realization came to me. This seemed crazy, but I knew where my father had gone when he died twelve years earlier. I can't say this tiny being was an embodiment of my dad, like a reincarnation; but my question got answered. I touched his nose. Mom smiled.

I said, "Thank you. You are blessed to have him."

"I know," she replied, smiling. As they walked off, a tear welled up.

I knew I was starting to come back to life.

BIOMEDICAL PROCESSES

Modern medicine is amazing. Sometimes I wish I had a mind that's more disciplined, more attuned to learning the "hard sciences." The few times I've read or studied anatomy and physiology, I've shaken my head in wonder. Advances in science have accelerated enormously since 1900, disproportionate to advances in the first several thousand years of man's history. I feel thankful that I'm still alive, because antibiotics and medical procedures saved my life. Public Health gives extended life to millions of us.

The single most important medical breakthrough about the plague came in 1894, when Alexandre Yelsin identified a bacillus responsible for that illness. Shortly before this, the third pandemic began in China in the 1860's. One researcher wrote: "The disease thereafter became endemic and throughout the 1880's slowly traveled eastward through provinces, reaching Canton in 1894." Because of the proximity, Hong Kong was hit in May and declared an "infected port." Within the next twenty years, bubonic plague spread from southern Chinese ports throughout the world, causing more than ten million deaths. The World Health Organization considered it active until 1959."[10] A Japanese research team headed by Dr. Kitasato Shibasaburo arrived in Hong Kong on June 12, 1894. Dr. Shibasaburo had studied with Dr. Robert Koch in Germany, who discovered the anthrax and tuberculosis bacilli and the serum for them. Dr. Shibasaburo grew the bacillus responsible for tetanus. He knew his stuff. Hong Kong British Colonial Surgeon and inspector of hospitals Philip Ayers gave the Japanese team full support. Alexandre Yersin, however, a lone Frenchman who had studied with Pasteur and had isolated the diphtheria exotoxin, received no such assistance. In four days he discovered the bacillus responsible for plague, wrote a brilliant report and helped create a serum which proved effective, though costly. After a dispute, the bacillus, Yersinia pestis, was named after him, but not until the 1940's.

Other significant research on fleas and the bacillus reveals interesting dynamics. Not all rodents carry deadly fleas, nor do all fleas carry the plague bacteria. When they do, fleabites are known to regurgitate 25,000 to 100,000 bacilli into the victim's tissue. Strangely, as white blood cells attack *Yersinia pestis* engulfing it and releasing killing enzymes, the plague bacillus uses two avoidance mechanisms. They not only protect it, but allow it to attach to white cells for transportation throughout the body, especially to the lymph nodes. Infection proliferates. Some have termed this the Microbial Dance of Death. Body temperature rises in an effort to "cook" the invader. If it survives this, infected lymph nodes show discoloration within three days. When this happens, the probability of mortality is 60 percent. DNA research from specimens has shown three types that mirror the pandemics, tracing their roots:

Antigua (Justinian's)

Medievalis (Black Death)

Orientalis (Last pandemic from China through the Pacific Rim).

From the 18th century on, villagers realized that when there was an epidemic of dead rats, people got sick and died. In 1898 this was shown to be more than an old wives' tale. It was proved that rats carry the flea that carries the bacteria.

The last major outbreak of the plague in the United States was in 1924 in Los Angeles, when thirty-one people died. In the 1960's, Vietnam reported 10,000 deaths a year from the plague through the 1970's. The tunnels, the rain, the dead bodies all facilitated a rise in the rat population. Then in September 1994 a form of the disease, pneumonic plague, struck in India. Contributing conditions were a recent earthquake, corpses of animals ignored due to Indian aversion to touching the dead, and Hindu customs preventing people from killing rats. Panic ensued with good reason. "When not treated, bubonic disease becomes systemic and affects the lungs and other vital organs; coughing spreads plague bacillus through the air. This virulent infection then spreads by droplet from person to person, and when inhaled, infects the lungs, causing pneumonic plague, which may cause death the first day of the infection."[11] The number of suspected cases was 4500, with 1000 diagnosed and approximately 234 deaths. Untimely response to critical indicators is responsible for the large number of deaths. Once again, economic and political factors kept those in charge from acting. The World Health Organization *Plague Manual* describes in detail the procedures to be undertaken when cases of plague occur in a given area. This information was not promptly utilized in India. So many died because once again, no one wanted to say, "It's here." The World Health Organization has recently categorized the plague as a re-emerging disease.

You may ask, "What about it is changing and adapting? In 1995, a strain of multidrug-resistant (MDR) Y. *pestis* was taken from a bubonic plague patient in Madagascar and was resistant to at least eight antimicrobials, including streptomycin, tetracycline, chloramphenicol, and sulfonamides." To date, this is the only documented case of MDR Y. *pestis*, although there is no systematic monitoring of resistance. It appears no one is watching it, really.

10 Chase, M.

11 Tysmans, J.B. Plague in India—1994 Conditions, Containment, Goals

DR. RED

Every time we spoke it seemed like there was something that he wanted to tell me. His poker face really wasn't. As the Chief of the Infectious Disease Team we connected right-off-the-bat. Once when he leaned close to me to check my breathing I told him he had bad breath. Smiling he looked right at me and said, "So do you." I can only imagine what was going through his mind: "There was a part of me that wished I could tell him what we suspected. His condition was so critical upon admission that I'm really surprised he survived. That bubo on his left inside thigh was very telling. When those occur the disease is fatal in 60 percent of cases. Somehow he made it, miraculously. Since he was delirious from fever (which is the body's way of cooking intruders to death), there was no way to find out what we were dealing with. So, we began tests, especially cultures, some of which took up to ten days to produce a result. In the meantime, just keeping him alive was the challenge. He wasn't eating solids and was losing weight rapidly. Infection, which is how the plague kills, was everywhere in his body. And pain, too. As he was hardly able to move, it was necessary to place a catheter in him. That had to hurt.

"We began treating for plague, but were waiting for tests to confirm that diagnosis. From the bubo we assumed this—no other disease produces that effect. Since the Middle Ages it has been the primary indicator. Immediately upon his arrival we started him on antibiotics. Prior to WW II there was no predictable treatment for the plague, really. His condition was advanced and precarious. Perhaps his good health got him to us rather than to the morgue. Observing him during Grand Rounds when so many doctors and students were discussing his case, I could tell he was not happy being the guinea pig. However, his overall attitude was amazing. Even though he could hardly move nor knew what would happen next, he did not complain. And the number of visitors was astounding. Several men came almost daily and there was an aura of peace and calm in that room. The RN in charge of daily care told me something else: he thanked the staff a lot. We really don't get much appreciation for what we do, but he was genuinely grateful, especially for the cleaning staff.

"When the diagnosis was confirmed, he became very interested in the plague, always asking questions. We had to do research to satisfy him: history of occurrence (in New Mexico as well as worldwide), diagnostic indicators, treatment, and prognosis.

"Something unusual was driving this guy. He was so weak, often talking gibberish, but lucid enough to keep us on our toes. But That talk about the presence of death got bothersome. So we had various chaplains stop by to see him. They reported that he was all right, in good spiritual condition, even brightening up their days. Feeling a satisfaction in treating someone does not happen around here that often. When he was moved to another room in the hospital the treatment team missed him; but were unusually pleased with the outcome. Indeed, with antibiotics and modern medicine he lived. That did not look like it was going to happen when he arrived."

Thanks, Doc.

A REAL TRAGEDY

Over three million people a year die of infectious disease on our planet. Probably that figure would be higher if accurate records were available. The bubonic plague claims only about 1,000 of us yearly, if that. In New Mexico only eight people died of plague in 2005, and sixteen in the United States as a whole. These are not just numbers. These were real people like you and me with families, children and stories of their own. With all of our advancements in science, we still can't stop this. However, research has opened up areas of inquiry once thought unconnected to infection. Now peptic ulcers and cervical cancer are showing themselves highly influenced by bacteria. Even some Alzheimer's patients have shown improvement when treated by antibiotics.

Scientists say bacteria are so important, that life on this planet would cease without them. Actually microbes may be the reason there is life at all on Earth. Apparently it was the microbes in the water that created oxygen that enabled our ancestors to generate themselves. Now that's amazing.

Not all bacteria are harmful. Physical health depends on the "good" ones. The immune system which keeps the equation balanced (as the Oracle told Neo in *The Matrix*) in our bodies, consists of the bacteria that enhance digestion and contribute positively to overall well-being. It is even being suggested that mental health (or not) could be a function of these critters. Yep, bugs can operate in the brain. Probiotics is the contemporary study of healthful, useful bacteria; and how they can be used to enhance our longevity. These have names like: 'L.reuteri, L casei, L.lactis, L.acidophilus, B.lactis, L.rhamnsus, B.bacterium longum, etc., and are available is cultures like yogurt, especially a product called kefir.

If you really, really want to see what could happen in a 21st century pandemic, watch the movie *Contagion*. It's all about compounding accidents, especially how environmental factors contribute directly: a bat defecated in a pig pen, then the pig was slaughtered, eaten, then the 'dark force' was in the human population. Though difficult to watch, there seemed to be truth in that tale. Mine is a small piece of the infectious disease story.

Now, what about Ebola?

THAT HAS TO BE WHAT HAPPENED!

Seems to me it was a beautiful day. Full summer had landed at 7300 feet on the Great Divide headed east out of Albuquerque. That's the point where the Estancia Valley really opens up to the plains. Some call it the high desert, but it's not because of the sand. There are a lot of trees up there. Big ones like the Ponderosa pines with long needles and trunks that can grow to be a couple of feet wide at the base. Some are so tall that if you take the time to look up, all you can say is "Wow!" Once I was in the Vatican gazing in wonder at the ceiling of the Sistine Chapel. If I didn't keep my balance I would have toppled over. Then I felt a tear trickling down my earlobe. The same thing can happen when gazing up at these magnificent trees. Being touched by such beauty is at once humbling and awesome. "Only God can make a tree."

Several years before this, my brother Dan and I were driving down the two-lane road to my home in a rainstorm. Not a hundred feet ahead of us lightning hit a behemoth of a tree. The ground shook like it does when an airplane breaks the sound barrier. Smoke was coming off it, and on the ground at the trunk we saw a blackened spot around an impression in the earth where the high voltage grounded. That smoky, burned smell filled our nostrils. It was not quite like being next to a barbecue, sweeter, like a sappy pine odor. Looking up, we saw that the bark had been split apart top to bottom, like a long knife had opened its skin. Innards exposed, airborne attackers would surely take her life in short order. Her majesty was humbled by the very nature she represented.

Sprinkled about are juniper trees with lovely bows for arms sprouting beautiful bluish berries that are used to make the liquor, gin. A walk through these woods is no easy matter, what with bushes between most of the trees. Called scrub oak by locals, they never seem to grow tall, but scratch as hikers wend their way around this, then that obstacle. Straight lines rarely exist in nature, the path being a lot like life. Of course, piñon pine trees are everywhere, producing the nuts available at grocery stores, or free for the taking from the trees. The nuts ripen and drop in the fall, just about the time the aspen trees go from green to golden yellow. Families who have lived in the area for a long time still take picnic meals and head for the hills, hoping to beat the squirrels to the cache. They know where to go, and it's not to the grocery store. No doubt an elder family member has been guiding the family to treasured spots for generations. A few roadside stands along old Route 66 still sell fresh piñon nuts that don't carry FDA stamps. Nobody worries about that.

It was early August, just prior to this time of year, when my friend Professor Joe, between semesters, made his quarterly visit to the Land of Enchantment. Having purchased acreage a few years earlier, my itinerant neighbor had returned for golf, exploring the flea markets, eating green chili enchiladas and spending long days on his soon-to-be hacienda. He works like a madman, driven to finish a project before dark stops him. Often, it's the only thing that can. This particular trip, the first week of August, 2006, ushered in a new arrival: a 1963 aluminum-skinned Airstream drag-behind trailer, tarnished by forty-three years of high-UV southwest sun. Right away after he had arrived he had gone on his usual scavenger hunt along the Mother Road (Route 66), headed east out of Edgewood. There, on the north side a few miles out of town at a dying trailer park, he discovered the trailer. Arriving back that day at my owner-built, six-sided home, he was ecstatic with the news of this steal of a deal. Now the question was, "How do we move her the twelve miles up here?" Fortunately, a neighbor, Little John (actually not so little), a jack-of-all-trades, was easily enrolled into the caper.

The next day, with air tanks to fill the tires, straps to secure any loose ends, along with jacks and timbers, we started his diesel pickup for the trip. As we headed down off the mountain, I shared the excitement of this adventure. Under the blazing hot sun with low humidity, cloudless blue sky and a supply of cold water, we worked like a seasoned team to resuscitate the antique.

With the trailer in tow, we slowly lumbered back up the mountain, well prepared, almost ready for a breakdown. We dared it to happen. Not infrequently, high energy and clear intention (plus preparation) can create a zone where things just fall into place. They did that day. With the radio playing old rock-and-roll through high-quality speakers, frequent checks on the "load," and an ace wheelman jamming the gears, we arrived safely with Professor Joe's treasure by mid-afternoon siesta time. However, no rest was to be had, yet. Backing in, blocking, even blessing the landing seemed like the dessert for our efforts.

Though clearly aged, the Airstream had no body damage of any consequence. Her casement windows were intact and would still open and close, and she still had the original rounded-around-the-top door, which to my mind resembled a Hobbit portal. She was just plain stout. Frankly, I could not wait to enter her. After leveling the trailer and thanking our moving-man neighbor, we sat our sweaty bodies down for a respite. We were happy guys. After a too-short rest, we dragged our old bones up in anticipation. Joe had even gotten a key for the working lock. Since he had inspected the beauty before purchasing it, I had not yet gone inside. Unbeknownst to me a centuries old killer lurked there.

Man, it was a treat to walk through that entry...like crossing a threshold into another world. Just across from the door was the plywood cabinetry, which was in pretty good shape. The unique locks were still in good working order. They look like a round white knob a couple of inches in diameter that you have to grab with a thumb and forefinger. As you twist it, the inner spring tightens and the catch releases—very ingenious. Below the upper cabinets on the wall across from the door and a little to the left was the still-functional divided aluminum sink. There was a small cutting board on one side with a just-big-enough finger-pull at one side. Curious, I lifted it and saw a fist-sized bundle of insulation, twigs and bits of rags. Obviously some critter(s) had set up a homestead, but that was Joe's problem.

Someone, probably years earlier, had painted the ceiling in the mini-living room to the right of the entry a gaudy mauve. There were seats along both sides under the colorful canopy, about six feet long and probably 30 inches deep with musty smelling cushions. Between them was a 24-inch walkway that could perhaps someday be used for places to sit or sleep. Walking back past the mini-kitchen area toward the rear of this coach, I spied a quite compact one-piece molded bathroom. All the way at the back was a cute little sink, above which was a three-foot-wide window—brush your teeth as you watch where you've been. With a compact shower and tub to the left and commode to the right, all of the necessary elements were in place for life on-the-road. Few cracks were visible, and to the casual observer (like my excited friend) all looked just "peachy." But being a guy who knows something about infrastructure, my concern was for things like:

Waterlines connected and not cracked?

Electrical wiring still usable? (And not chewed through by rodents?)

Propane line secure and leak-free?

Oh, and those soft spots in the floor. Has it rotted out?

However, Joe was like a kid with $5.00 let loose in a candy shop. It was not the time to address these questions that for me were at the heart of the trailer's functioning. In vehicles like this there are no odometers, but she showed some signs of her age, and obviously needed someone to love her back to life. My pal was the right guy for the job, all right. He and I share a passion for resuscitation of things others see little hope in. That's why we like flea markets; but variously one or the other of us needs to call a halt when an interesting piece is well beyond its shelf life or would take too much time or money to regenerate. This was not one of those. We could have been heroes on PAWN STARS.

She was a beauty for sure. In her prime she had been the queen of the highway, not unlike a model or movie star. Well, that might be a bit much. To friend Joe she still held that place of prestige, and he was damned proud to have rescued this damsel. That's one of his admirable characteristics: he likes to help others, with women high on the list.

After the once-over on the interior, we commenced a dust-and-clean of cabinets and drawers. That's when it happened, I believe. Like an unsuspecting prey who stepped into a trap nature had set into motion centuries ago, I made a contact that would dramatically alter my life.

In the short corridor between the kitchen area and the bathroom at the rear was a set of four or five drawers on the left side. Opening the top one, I saw another bundle of debris made up of pieces of insulation, weeds and twigs. Clearly this was another rodents' nest. Looking closer at it, I saw some of the residents were at home. With no hesitation, having work gloves on, I seized the comfy little abode as gently as possible, walked to the open door and placed it outside a few feet away. No thought was given to any repercussions; I simply thought this was a kinder approach than a heavy-handed disposal. That compassionate act was no guarantee of a positive outcome for me.

That moment was very costly. How often do we hear the story of a driver looking away from the road at a critical moment and causing a major accident. If I'd only known, I might have done something different.

I had no immediate sense of an intruder, as an infected plague flea made its way up my left arm, biting and regurgitating thousands of bacteria into my body. I slept all right that night, ate breakfast the next day, and continued helping clean up the Airstream. However, for some reason I couldn't understand, in the afternoon nausea overcame me and I vomited in the bushes in the shadow of that beautiful death-trap.

WHAT WERE YOU DOING UP THERE IN THE FIRST PLACE?

Cities, large or small, have never felt right to me. Obviously, not everyone is this way, but I'm one of those who had to "get out of Dodge." I can survive amid buildings and neighborhoods where there are enjoyable distractions available. But when all the noise evaporates, as quiet descends, there's not much soul in concrete, steel and asphalt. Once upon a time I'd found that peace in the woods. Just like one's "first," I remember that trip. Etched in my neurotransmitters is the picture of my high school pals and me camping out of a four-door 1956 Ford in Michigan on a weekend in 1963. Our campsite overlooked a lake, and the three or four of us had the time of our lives.

Now it was 1994, and my father had died, gone to that mysterious place called the afterlife. I missed him. Then something strange happened to me. I had lived in Albuquerque for 14 years and was well into owning my second home, but city life suddenly lost its appeal. Perhaps my own mortality became clearer, as I realized there was less time ahead than behind. I was 48. There were things I wanted to do in the time I had left. Over the years since arriving in New Mexico, camping trips and drives through the country had piqued my interest in rural living. "For Sale" signs always got my attention, and I had anxiously explored some of these properties. More than once when I looked at land to buy, the memory of that summer in Montana returned.

Jeanette and I had sold our furniture, packed our tools and our meager belongings (plus our faithful dog, Buck) in a pick-up truck in Ohio, cashed in our savings accounts and headed west. It was 1974, and not unlike early settlers, we hit the road headed for ten acres of Big Sky Country we'd purchased the previous summer while on our honeymoon. Arriving west of Missoula in June, we set up a large tent and proceeded to hew a small log cabin out of the wilderness for ourselves in Frenchtown, up Houle creek.

What a delicious time we had as newlyweds meeting kindly old timers and others like ourselves who were having yet another adventure of a lifetime. Dan Rose and Muffin were like an uncle and aunt; they took us under their wings, no doubt reliving their own past through our expectant future. He was an engineer, or "hoghead" on the Northern and Pacific railway. As an old cowboy he showed me how to break horses in between mending fences and keeping his appointments for chemotherapy treatments. Diagnosed with cancer within the first year I'd met him, that man showed me how to face death.. Right up to the end, he kept bargaining, *"If I can just hang on 'til the spring and see the foals drop."* He didn't. I couldn't go to the funeral. Instead I went to the corral and talked to the horses. They listened and seemed to understand. Even now, thirty-some years later, I miss that man.

Then there was that alcoholic reprobate Chuck Dawson, who worked ranches, poached deer and lived an old cowboy's life as if he were surviving on the frontier, which he was. Once he had to go to court for a speeding ticket. He said that the judge asked him why he didn't have a driver's license. All he could say was "Hell, yer Honor, I ain't got no birth certificate 'cause I was born in a log cabin in the Bitterroot Mountains." That poor judge just shook his head and dismissed the charges. Those were carefree days, for sure.

Years later, 1994, I longed for a similar simple life in the high country of the Land of Enchantment away from the lights of Albuquerque. There comes a time, infrequently, when one gets a glimmer of something just over there on the horizon. Like when a few pieces start to fall together in a jigsaw puzzle, or that intuitive moment during a word puzzle when one word makes all the difference in finishing it. That's what it felt like. Five years earlier a friend had rented a small house east and south of town. To relocate, he'd organized a moving party on a weekend and I was part of it. After that I'd visited him and his companion, Dusty D dog, several times. He's such a character: a loner who worked the phones to raise money for various causes, skimming a bit off of the top for living expenses. Over the years he has struggled with military-related PTSD, yet been a consistent brother-inquirer into soul/spirit matters, always bringing me a new twist on some old theme. However, more than anything else, it was the quiet of his new location that I enjoyed so much.

Without conscious thought I took a spring afternoon trip in the direction where my friend had lived. (He'd since moved back to the city–the hassle of daily commutes overrode the pleasure of solitude.) Apparently following an unconscious suggestion, the truck took a left onto a dirt road near his old place. (Somewhere between "Drive" and "Park" on the steering column must be "Intuitive." Everyone has this attribute, but little did I know a vehicle might possess it.) This was not some potholed, unkempt lane. There was room for two vehicles to easily pass each other, but I saw none all afternoon. Trees of all descriptions as well as bushes lined both sides, and there was a drainage swale clear of blockage. Somebody was maintaining this place. Though just off of a paved county road, it seemed remote, but not quite isolated.

By chance, I'd entered my future homestead area. And it felt that way: no homes (or trailers) in sight, good solar visibility available, hawks chasing other critters across the sky, rabbits hurrying out of the way, with coyotes and bears probably spying on me. Then, lo and behold, a hand-made For Sale sign showed itself, tacked to a tree up on the right. I couldn't believe it: no doubt a sign from the Creative Intelligence. I copied the number and managed to drive home without breaking the sound barrier. A calm voice answered when I called. That phone, that evening was my best friend. My excitement was running high, as if a long-sought-after prize was within reach. It was all I could do to keep from blurting out, "I want that land!"

We all have wants. People want to lose weight, get a new car, a better job, girlfriend (or boyfriend) or whatever. In a training session a long time ago, a trainer said to me, "There's not a lot of power in what you want; it's what you are committed to that matters." In my best questioning voice I inquired, "What is a commitment?" He asked me to visualize a plate of bacon and eggs. Then he said: "The chicken was involved, and the pig was committed." Oh.

It also means persistence. One of my mentors is a writer who's been picking up his pencil for sixty years, every day, no matter what. Not surprisingly, he's published books and screenplays. Another friend, Juan, a martial arts teacher, told me, " I look for opportunities to engage in Tae Kwon Do." That kind of single-minded focus has mostly eluded me. The one thing that has escaped me much of my life is something to be wholeheartedly dedicated to. Perhaps the fulfillment of this vision of owning a property outside the city would be that.

Tom, the man who answered my call, explained that his wife had owned the property for thirty years, that the road was maintained by the County, but most importantly, that they would carry a land contract with a minimal down payment. Containing my excitement, I set a meeting time with Tom for the next weekend. Seven days dragged by. Finally he met me at the appointed time the next Saturday, under that For Sale sign (that hung high on a tree) for a walk around the property.

Out there, away from the noises of the city, the silence was all-pervasive. It's said that there are three great mysteries: air to the birds, water to the fish, and man to himself. The "quiet" has got to be another one for us. When it is found and embraced there's something refreshing, even in only a moment's worth of an inhalation. You take a deep breath and say, "AHHHH."

Next I noticed the sun. Since my construction apprenticeship was with a solar energy builder, the position of this land allowed direct access to *El Sol*. Textbooks, magazines, and websites abound which describe the simple process of erecting a building in relationship to the sun's east/west pathway. All a constructor has to do is face windows to the south (in the northern hemisphere), insulate well, perhaps add a greenhouse, and voilà! Free heat! Without much trouble, I could visualize my home right before my very eyes: an enclosed entry on the north side at the end of the driveway from the road opens into an airlock storage. From there one moves into the main living space through a hand-carved main door, not unlike an oversized castle entry. (I remember walking through one at the castle on the hill in Salzburg, Austria). Fantasy was alive and well that day.

Just south of where we parked, Tom and I moved quickly onto my imagined land of Oz. Understandably he lagged behind a bit. I was the one champing at-the-bit. As we made our way around the underbrush, he slowed, then pointed out a potential building site that had a ledge behind it. Though it was a prospective clearing and was interesting, there was much more to see. Somewhere during the first 15 minutes I sneaked in the all-important question, "How much are you asking?"

"$28.5" was the simple answer.

Feigning a modicum of stoicism, I kept quiet as he continued. "The property is surveyed into two pieces. This one is 1.3 acres, and the adjoining one is 1.75."

We stopped in a clearing overlooking a small ridge. I looked directly at him, an arm's distance away. "Would you take $3,000 down and carry the rest on a land contract?" I asked in what I hoped was a mature tone, trying not to sound like I was begging.

His "*Yes*" lit me up like a Christmas tree. My hand shot across to his, we shook, smiled and finished our tour. The rest of the show-and-tell excursion was whipping cream on the strawberry shortcake on that afternoon. He said that he knew an escrow company who could handle the transaction. On Monday a week later we met at the appointed place and time, signed papers, and I handed over the check. I became a landowner, steward to my vision, caretaker of my future home in the mountains.

At that time I was renting a room from a friend in Albuquerque. Within a week of closing the deal, I set up a camping spot on an easily cleared overlook, implementing a long-thought-through plan. Now it was only work that stood between me and my dream fulfilled. And work was something that I not only knew how to do, but enjoyed. Bringing a home of my own design out of the ground was the next adventure.

Within a week of signing the papers, a friend of a friend, Buzz, helped me lay out a conventional rectangular plot for a home. Something wasn't right about it, though. As I walked around the string lines where the walls were to be built, then stepped inside to sit in the once-and-future living room an idea came to me. *It's my house---do something different.* Having worked in Navajo land where homes were six or eight sided (called a Hogan), the vision of a mountain 'Hogan' presented itself to me. Often I'm not sure if I'm the inventor of something, or if that thing wanted to come-to-be, with my own self as the vehicle. In any event the commitment was hatched and the 'case-was-afoot' as Sherlock Holmes would have said.

In September of 1997 the power pole was planted. In August of 2000 all bills were paid off by a home-owners loan. I took up residence. My mom Ruth used to say that I never finished things. She died in 1999 leaving me $10,000. That money was used to put finishing touches on my home. Poetic justice, somehow. Thanks mom!

FAMILY MATTERS

Being a loner has a good side: it's a way to avoid Other People's Bullshit. However, when I was in the hospital dying, it was my brothers and sisters I wanted to be with me. Only brother Dan, who lives close by, came almost daily. Why didn't the other five ask if I needed them? Maybe it was because I didn't ask them, or that my loner ways were coming back to haunt me.

But let's face it, living the way I have, some days loneliness is my companion. There is a price for everything; was I paying it now? Early in life, I, like most people, escaped into my own head space. Over a period of time, even dealing with one's own can of crap can wear thin. I didn't become psychotic; I just learned that I had to be OK with myself. That's a life task.

As a kid with so many of us crammed into a three-bedroom home, my own little world became sacrosanct—I didn't want anyone invading my territory. But when I was in that hospital dying, I wanted them by my side. I was really scared. Now, looking back at myself, I can see why it didn't happen.

Growing up in a small suburban house with six siblings and a set of parents, all using one bathroom, there wasn't much privacy. Even my mom would lock herself in the bathroom to escape the din. The little kids would cry and pound on the door. We older ones would pick them up and console them. Little did we realize that her time-out saved us from her pent-up frustration. My time-out, as a pre-teen kid, began as a morning paper-delivery boy. When I got up at 5:00 a.m. with nobody around, the world seemed to be mine.

The summer trips to the swimming pool ten miles east provided adventure, too. Then there were the bike odysseys with pals to the strawberry fields, where we'd make ten cents per quart for picking; and paid ourselves the bonus of a bellyful. That was the season to be outside, away from the crowd. I still love summers, being out of doors. Back then, after babysitting for mom in the mornings, I earned my freedom. In my own mind I was an explorer. That's stayed with me. When I couldn't go outside, I went inside myself.

Years later, lying in that plague bed, alone, drugged-up, with medical people in and out all of the time, inside I went. In there, some days it was moment-by-moment catastrophe waiting to happen: too many fears. Isn't it strange how thoughts and feelings tend to play off of each other? Once on a roll with either, they suck the other one in, and downhill I would go, headed for the worst. What helped me back to some sanity, even provided needed distraction were memories of my family. Everyone has a personal connotation for the word for that special group of kin, though there's no real definition of it.

We don't get to choose our blood type, nor who transported it to us, nor those with whom we share it. Some say, at an esoteric level, we choose our parents with accompanying life style before birth. That's an interesting conjecture, but I'd rather stay in this here, earthly reality for my inquiry. Getting lessons in this life is hard enough. Certainly no human being is exempt from familial issues in the bag we carry. For starters, parents bring their sack full, which they received from their caretakers. Talk about hand-me-downs! More like clothes from a cousin—some fit and some don't; but you still have to wear them. We all have to learn our life lessons.

The school of hard knocks is a rough teacher. No one escapes that one either, nor the unfinished dramas of childhood. Yet some still succeed, in spite of them, or because of them. Who decides? How does one person growing up in horrible circumstances fail miserably, while another in the exact same situation makes it? Most would shake their heads and say there's no way to know. But there is a place to go to unravel the mystery. Like Ellery Queen, I was a detective, driven to understand my own family. The path took me to social sciences.

The Department of Family Studies is where I ended-up in the mid-80's when I returned to graduate school. I'd found a place to begin the search. Looking back, it doesn't surprise me that I wound up in that academic area, nor that I got good grades. There was plenty of grist for that mill in my own personal history, and grind away it did. Facing the consequences of my ordinal position as oldest ("Who's in charge here?"), addressing an intergenerational inheritance of alcohol dependence (both Mom and Dad were children of alcoholics) was not fun. But I sure learned a thing or two. Those lessons were taken back to the substance abuse treatment center where I worked full time while in school. As a counselor-in-training, I learned skills, then practiced them with patients' family members on Family Day.

Adolescent patients' siblings, parents and others came for eight hours of emotional meat grinding on Thursdays. We were implementing Multiple Family Group Therapy, doing cutting-edge work, which was exciting. Imagine thirty or forty people in one large room going at it with four or five staff members, focusing on unresolved issues which most likely had landed the kids in that residential hospital. Couples' dysfunction, parenting styles, divorces, and adult addiction, all became visible. Our team was so skilled and professional that progress was evident in many lives, including our own.

There are enough examples of this kind of work to fill a book, which someone has probably written. To begin with, to do that job, a major shift in thinking was necessary: there was no *one* patient. The family as a whole was the target of the therapeutic process. Having a clear understanding of my own history was both a shock and an asset. One of the double-edged swords of existence: Hate your parents, love your parents. I was lucky to have gotten good ones, though that realization has come to me slowly over the years.

Since my mom, Ruth, had to raise seven kids, feed nine people every day and manage a household, there wasn't much one-to-one time with her. I remember that at the age of four or five, I was her "go-fer." Even at that age I was already "parentized."

My dad, Mason, was a WWII veteran, no doubt suffering from PTSD, and was emotionally distant during most of my childhood. He didn't talk much. One day I realized he didn't say, "I love you" much. But he showed his love through his actions. I never went hungry and never lacked clothing or shelter. I got to attend schools that were adequate or better. I was force-fed discipline (with the Bolo paddle on occasion), taught respect, and shown a spiritual path. I received good guidance through tough love, as well. Dad and his four younger brothers were scrappy Irishmen from the south side of Toledo who knew how to fight and survive. The way they lived every day prepared them for war; Toledo's "Purple Gang" kept boys on their toes. So when he went to war, he was ready to deal with the Germans and the Japanese.

His dad, Grandpa Lou, was a real drunk whose "sainted" wife, Ethel (Dad's mom), died young in the 1930's when my dad was in his early teens. Alone, Lou tried to raise the boys, but actually they were mostly farmed out to extended family members. There were plenty of stories about that. After the war, in 1946, when Dad was 29, he met and married my mother, Ruthie, who was 19 at the time and from the east side of Toledo. Amazingly (well, maybe not), I arrived that year, also.

Mom had six older siblings: Lavona, Eulela, Lyle, Katherine (Kate), Jim, and Mary. Her dad, Albert, was a drunk. There must have been a lot of that around then. Lavona (we called her Aunt Onea), helped start Al-Anon in Toledo because her husband, Ike (a good name for a drunk), had a bad drinking problem. So did Aunt

Kate's husband, Uncle Carl. They were my godparents. Obviously, with this much alcoholism in my immediate family, I was steeped like a tea bag in the "sauce." It's called "pickled" for a reason.

Two of Dad's brothers were alcoholics. A third, Fred, probably was too. Somehow Dad and Wayne escaped that designation. Liquor was the social lubricant at family functions like baptisms, birthday celebrations, weddings and the infamous Christmas Eve party. At that holiday gathering a good fistfight was always on the agenda; there was no silent night. Ruthie complained a lot, to which Dad laughed, explaining it as "brothers blowing off steam." Maybe so, but the odor was tainted. It's just the way they grew up–the way they were trained, if you will. We're all programmed, one way or another.

Families, like all systems, operate by rules. The most powerful are those unspoken. In school as well as the popular literature of that time, it was suggested that substance-dependent families ran themselves by three main ones: Don't talk, Don't feel, Don't trust. Two out of three and you win (or lose). Mother owned and dished out all of the emotion; actually she was histrionic. Who wouldn't be, living her job description? Over the years I've discovered that I am my mother's son, having fed at the trough of those emotions. That's probably one reason why I was a good family therapist: no one could out do, out think or out-emote me. I'd been there all right. Affective intensity has been my normal operating state, over which I have had to get. It's one of those hand-me-downs I've outgrown, for my own good, and the world's.

Researchers say that the most enduring memories have the strongest emotions attached, and that makes sense. That's the basis of PTSD. No wonder this mind of mine is so full of powerful memories. Another well imprinted operating principle connected to emotional survival in our family is "Quick wit connected to acerbic tongue." It was deeply embedded in the Mason/Ruth culture and still is to this today. When I get with any of the six others and the "smart-ass" comes at me, I have to remind myself, "Oh, I'm with my family–not everyone talks this way." Without saying what is on one's mind, a sarcastic retort or smart-aleck remark pops up, which is really an effort to connect or communicate. That's what we learned: "Don't talk directly!" This is not to say we weren't close, or didn't care for each other. We do.

Over the years we've been able to be more direct about what we say and how we feel. Recently, after more than forty years of marriage, sister Bonnie's husband, Jack, dropped over dead from a heart attack at 62. He was a really good man. A couple of months after the wake-like family gathering, I spoke to her on the phone. Softly I asked how she was doing with her grieving. Dead silence. After a bit I said, "Are you still there?" A sob came back at me, and I started to cry, too. This touches me, even now. The depth of feeling often lies quietly until jerked out of its hiding by a needed connection. I've been there, on the need-to-be-connected-to end. That's a lesson from the plague.

Still, even though Dan got my plague-ridden body to the hospital, visited daily, and baby sister Mary kept in touch with the medical staff, I missed the others. Having been gone for more than forty years from Ohio, 1200 miles west, it wasn't like crossing town for them to come and sit at my bedside. But I hadn't disappeared from their lives. During my hiatus, I made trips to Ohio almost yearly, especially when our parents were still living.

Actually, the summer before the plague adventure, I spent three months in the Midwest heat being cooked to well done by the humidity. I'd forgotten that part. Living in the dryness of the desert, it wasn't a hankering for 80 percent humidity that drew me there, nor memories of my old Ohio home. Sister Kitty, the exact middle of the troupe, needed her kitchen remodeled. The suburban brownstone was in need of an update. Not trusting unknown workmen, she called on me. I was enrolled, called off of the bench for active duty. Kiwi, as she is affectionately called, has assumed the mom duties; and I got marching orders.

When our mom passed in '99, my baby sister called, saying, "Now we are orphans." I think that realization solidified our team. Her passing was not unexpected. Six years earlier Mom had a heart attack on the operating table when physicians were working on her for a diabetes-related leg problem. She ultimately lost one of her lower limbs. Undaunted, she persevered long past her life expectancy. Doctors predicted two years. She showed them, and us. (Could it be I get my tendency toward defiance from her?) A stroke finally got her, and somebody had to be the one in charge after her demise. Kiwi got the job. The others of us have recognized it, agreeing that it's OK.

Years earlier, on a visit to New Mexico, Kiwi had seen the home I'd built and knew I could do the job she had in mind. Since I was available, I went, figuring it would be an easy job that would take a month or so. I loaded my tools, and a long, uneventful drive put me in Columbus in early June. That's just in time for the hot, humid summer. Little did I know until I got there, that the "little" job would turn into three months. But that was typical for me–I always underbid jobs. Special Corian countertops took six weeks to deliver from time of order. GRRR! Then there was the new oak floor to install. I saw I was going to be there the whole summer, which I was.

Coming from desert dryness, I did not greet sweltering heat with enthusiasm. With old cabinets removed and new ones ordered, the real work began. Of course the walls weren't straight and nothing was square. Frustration sat me down more than once before my tools went airborne. But on the positive side, together Kiwi and I created little touches that made her happy: special wall tiles that reminded her of a little town in France, a handmade wine rack above the stove, and storage shelves for the pantry. Seeing her joy made the job worth it. All the non-work time spent with siblings and their thirteen children was such a treat, as well. August is my birthday month and we had a great party to celebrate it. I got to feel special, dancing with the younger children, and spinning my sisters to old rock and roll songs.

The following summer, one week before the plague struck, all five siblings came to New Mexico for my 60th birthday. We'd never all been together in my home. There was a crowd, but I was in heaven. And Dan and Patricia got married that week, too. The service was held at a park near the reservation where she grew up. For months before the service they had been searching for someone to officiate. At the time Dan announced that they were getting hitched, I said I knew someone who could do it...me. He didn't know that six years earlier, at the millennium, I had gotten a certification as a real, honest-to-god minister. One of the changes I had wanted to make was a move into more spirituality. Morris, a friend whose connection to the eternal I admired, suggested that I search the Internet for resources. Lo and behold, a church in California, of course, offered a valid ministerial license for the asking. I did. They granted it. We all tend to think that something from the outside will make a difference on the inside. In our culture, the belief is that more possessions, better partner, bigger house, more education, credit cards or a certificate on the wall (obtained online), will finally make life better. But it got the job done for Dan and Pat. I was very honored. That's the only wedding I've ever done. A few shook their heads at the situation, especially Bonnie.

The oldest sister, Bonita Louise, affectionately known as Bon-Bon (the *n* is silent), married Jack, her college sweetheart, in 1971. They were happy. With a touch of the demure, at Dan's service, she offered her insight and advice to the couple: "I'm not sure I have much to say. Jack is such a good man. We just work at life together. I can be pretty outspoken, and he lets me, until he gets enough. Then he takes a weekend with his buddies. All of us sisters are close, so I'd say talk to your family about stuff and take their advice. I'm happy for you."

That's always been her way: brief. Short (so's she), to the point, sure of herself when she speaks. But always hidden, waiting to pop out, is a bit of humor or irony. We go back a long ways, more history together than anyone else in each others' lives, now that Mom and Dad have passed over. My earliest, clearest memory was Mom asking me to get a diaper so she could change Bon. The next was when our little family lived in the country near Lake Erie at Mominee Town. Actually it was just a church, rental house and cemetery. That's where we met a Catholic priest, Bernadine Rapinsky, OFM. (That stands for "Order of Friars Minor," meaning Franciscan.) Known to us as Father Butch, he and Dad liked to play golf and talk about Christianity.

There is a family story about how my little sister, in the summer, liked to take her clothes off and run through the graveyard. Three-year-olds do things unaware of prevailing conventions. On more than one occasion Father Butch brought her home. Somewhere along the way she learned to keep her pants on; and raised two great kids. She is a good human being. We have grown closer as I've looked at myself and been more open to my family, which I thought I'd escaped in 1974. One can never really do that. There's always Mother's Day and Father's Day to provide a jolt to the psyche. Bonnie and Jack forged a good life together. All four of my sisters married really solid men: good fathers as well as providers.

We brothers have not done so well, except number three of the seven, Timothy. He had blond hair and a slight build, and when he was a kid we called him "Skinny" (which he is definitely *not*, now). We all found out what a 'colic' was from him. His hair would never part; it went three directions at the top on the back of his head. He learned from his two older brothers the art of the quick retort to defend himself. As the oldest, I may have had something to do with that. That mind connected to this mouth was a virtual Claymore sword that was swung at others. Of course, as oldest I tried to inflict my will on Tim one too many times. We shared a bedroom, so occasionally when the lights went out, and we'd had a bit too much sugar before retiring, pillows would fly. Tickling was my "one-up" since I was physically bigger, and he would squirm so, yelling for "Mom!" That was my form of torment, always good as a threat, but never torture (I don't think so, anyway). We rolled around in snowball fights sometimes ending in tears, but we were never violent. He attended a rival co-ed high school in Toledo, so that contention provided lots of chances for witty repartee.

He resembles our father: mostly a quiet guy unless provoked, then cynicism flows. He's Christian (Catholic) to the bone (or soul), and an excellent father and husband with two granddaughters. A tenacious employee, he worked one job forever, retiring from the state of Ohio healthcare system as a Bureau chief.(That always reminds me of a chest of drawers.) My favorite remembrance is when he returned home, on leave from the Army in 1971. That was shortly after Jeanette and I had married. We fancied ourselves as jet setters, driving a Triumph TR-6 sports car. Loaning it to him, we felt good and so did he. Such a little thing, but it stayed with me. After his visit he went back to Germany, then transferred out of missile silos to a unit doing drug and alcohol counseling. (Ironic, given our family history.) That education may have saved him a degree majoring in substance abuse. Like most men, he keeps his own counsel and our phone conversations are few and far between, not unlike my dad and his brothers. Though he lives in the Columbus area where three of our sisters reside, they complain that they rarely get to see him. However, while I was hospitalized in my plague drama, he did ring me up. I don't remember much of that chat, except that he made a remark that made me chuckle. And of course I remember that he cared enough to call.

Another sister, Theresa, number five sibling, also contacted me. If any of us could be twins, we are the two. There is an unspoken affinity between us. Were I to have been born female in our family, I have no doubt I'd have been like her. Raising five healthy, honorably principled children, she is deeply spiritual, gentle, with a blessed dose of compassion. We don't communicate much, either, but when we connect, it's like good friends picking up right where we left off. There isn't much small talk; we get to heart-felt matters about our lives quickly.

All four of my sisters share an unusual bond. Several times a year they get together for a "girls weekend." As it so happened, probably ten years ago, I made a trip to Ohio that coincided with their scheduled gathering. They granted me the special status of "honorary sister" and I got to hang out with them. Lightheartedness prevailed. We all love to joke and laugh. One of the family stories we often recount is a "Comedy Central" moment: Something generated an out-of-control laughing spree, and one of them lost control of her bladder and wet her pants. That story brings a smile to me.

Now that I look back, there was no need for them to be at my bedside. Being in my heart, they truly were with me so.

THE MONK

Dozing off one evening after a bland hospital meal, I heard the oversized door open slowly. Its tell-tale squeak always gave away an intruder. "Weedhopper, are you in there?"

There's only one person who calls me that—a variation on "Grasshopper" from an old TV show. It had been a long day of visitors, ten to be exact, so another one wasn't really welcome. However, I got energy together for this one, whom I treasured. Not only a friend, but also a spiritual guide had made his way to me.

Years earlier we'd met in a seminar, taking training hours to maintain our professional licenses. Sitting next to each other, then, I opened my journal, which had been book marked with an embossed picture of the Buddha. "Ah, the Bude," he mused, nodding his head with a hint of a smile. There was the making of something inviting in his voice. His eyes said, *"Look here"* as he opened his book to reveal a similar icon. "Yes, sir" I whispered as the trainer looked askance at us. When the instructor announced that it was time for a break, we both headed for the coffee table, grabbed a cup and a chocolate chip cookie. As we moved toward the south terrace an early morning chill greeted us, which was a relief from the high-desert heat of summer. We sat down on a knee-high stone wall to the left of a set of beautifully hand-carved exterior wood doors. We felt comfortable being together.

"So you recognize the picture of the Buddha, eh?" I said.

"Oh, yah. If I ever meet that guy I swear I'll kill him!" blurted my coffee companion.

"Why in the world would you do that?"

"Because this life thing is about getting your own lessons— everybody's gotta figure out their own path. Outside help, even wizards, can only point the way, not do it for us. People attribute too much to the guru. Somebody says they've got the answer, walk away. He might have found a way for himself, but you'll pay one-way-or-the-other for thinking he's got it."

This was real news. Ever since I could remember there was something outside of me—parents, extended family members, teachers, God, church, adults in the neighborhood—who seemed to be in charge: teaching me, inflicting discipline, correcting me, basically, showing me their way. I was irritated. No one had ever been as direct as this guy, telling me about "inside growth," following an inner voice, finding peace with myself through compassion to others. I'd been raised Catholic, with the New Testament and church shoved into every orifice, almost. It seemed like I never really had any choice; it was their way or the highway. But their way wasn't my way; yet I didn't really know my way–I just didn't want to do it their way. Could this be the source of my "defiant disorder"? Chances are that I am not alone in this reaction.

Then he said that there are clearly marked paths that can be taken, including a spiritual one. I had tried for years to find it, but couldn't adapt anyone else's as my own. Here this peaceful, smiling fellow was telling me that I had to forge my own. At one point he told me some about his life, including that he was an ordained Buddhist Monk. "Come on" I said. "You're married, you work in prisons, and you're a monk? Plus you swear a lot."

"Forget about all of that," he said. "You've been trying to do this thing other people's ways. You don't need faith in some god, sitting on some throne up there in the clouds, who's ready to fry your ass. Truthfully, you need to get busy, pal!" He stopped, then took a sip from the paper cup he held in his hands, like a treasure. It seemed as if he were not really talking to me, but to the cup. Did it taste that good, or was that a strategy to see if I was listening? I was. But get busy at what? That's what I'd asked myself my whole life. People said about me, "He's got a lot of talent and energy. Someday, by golly, he'll be a real house afire when he figures out what to do with it." Here that was, in my face, again. Remember? Carl said that I have a message to carry, the Vets said to quit whining and get on with life. Even the housekeeper suggested that I have something yet to do this lifetime. One of my teachers once told me: "If one person calls you a horse's ass, forget it. If two do, go get fitted for a saddle." Some guys need four messages before they listen up.

"Don't be so dense, Weedhopper," the timid monk unloaded on me. "This world is butt-deep in suffering. You're a helper! Get over your resentments. Show them the way out, for Christ's sake."

Now, I've been hit over the head before, but some of us are a little denser than others. Waking up is double-edged. It's sort of like getting something nice that you like; then you have to take care of it. Buy a car, get insurance, pay for gas, deal with other boneheads on the highway; or just walk, perhaps hitchhike your way through life. Choose! Now you got the message. Be accountable!

"Sorry" he said, "I don't think you have a choice...you know what you have to do, don't you?" He was right. He left me to think about it as he got up and wandered over to a nearby flowerbed. He bent over, closed his eyes and seemed to go into a trance, breathing in the aroma of one particular rose. I expected him to return and sit with me, but no, he walked back into the seminar. I was left there to ponder the salt he'd shoved into the wound I'd carried for years. "Get over the resentment?" "Show them the way out?"

He had also said something to the effect that I didn't have to do anything about it. "Just be willing. The Creative Intelligence will put you to work when you're ready." *What is that?* I thought. I'd been taught "cognitive reorganization," heard "Plan your work...work your plan." Look forward into the future and lay-out activities. Now I'm just supposed to be willing? The rest of the morning session went in one ear and out the other as I jotted notes to myself about our conversation.

When the lunch break came, we both moved together without speaking to the restaurant. An affable waitress showed us to a quiet, out-of-the-way booth. When we were seated, the monk asked for an iced tea, then again shocked me by ordering a huge hamburger with everything on it.

"I thought monks were vegetarians," I said.

"There you go, again, laying your well-thought-through opinions on others. It's my gut and karma, not yours. Worry about what you're going to put in you; and who's paying for this meal, as I have no money."

"Oh, you're expecting me to buy?" I said.

"You want something from me, so you ought to pay for it. Suppose what we talk about is how to change your little life? Wouldn't that be worth the price of some dead cow?"

"So how do you know this is going to be life-altering?"

"Because you want it to be. You make a commitment right now that this chat will alter your whole existence and it will. Says who? You do, if you say so. Is my word that powerful? In your own life it is. Who else is in charge of you? Sit with that, I gotta pee."

While he was gone I was befuddled. Of course what he said was true, but I hadn't always lived that way. I'd rather blame others for damned near everything; and I couldn't seem not to. I knew that wasn't very mature. Sometimes I'd catch myself before I actually voiced my opinion, but the blame was in my mind, all the same. Then I thought of a plan to see what this guy was really about. If I was buying, I was going to get my money's worth.

Sliding back into the booth, he commenced the interrogation. He told me that he'd lived in Florida for quite a while before moving to Wyoming to take a job at a prison in a small town, then to New Mexico. Five years ago back in the Sunshine State, he had studied various religions in an attempt to connect more deeply to that Source, the Creative Intelligence. His mentor was a monk who directed the educational process and found a way to grant him college credit for his studies. Understandably, the new monk became a Buddhist and was eventually ordained. Along the way he had to let go of a promising musical career but continued his serious interest in golf. Apparently he was close to becoming a pro when he got the "word"' (a message he received intuitively) that he was supposed to carry "the message" instead. Now he chases the little white balls around on weekends. Buddhism and golf–an interesting combination.

Since it was a tee-shirt day when we met that summer, he was headed across the street that afternoon for 18 holes. He was not a tall fellow and not particularly muscular; I could see him succeeding at hitting par. Over dessert he said," My concentration on the game has gotten better since I quit drinking twenty-five years ago. Meditation helps me cut out distractions, too."

Quickly I chimed in, "I've been sitting on-and-off for a few years too–I pray for those suffering."

He replied, without a moment's hesitation, "From the news accounts, your prayers don't seem to be working." It came out the side of his mouth, sarcastically.

"Well, I...," I stammered, trying to explain what I am sure he already knew.

"Maybe you should pray for your own suffering ass, pal," he not so politely upbraided me.

There wasn't much I could say at that point. Though I had the illusions of success: a home, vehicles, and credit cards, something was missing. And not just a cute gal I could play house with two or three times a week. He was right-on about my suffering. I'd heard that "pain is given, suffering is optional," but how does one accomplish that shift? Webster says to suffer is "to endure or bear up under." Why is it that physical sensations of hurt can pass, but the remnants can go on for years, even unnoticed at the conscious level. That's suffering. It's so true of losses, especially. It didn't matter what kind: passing of a loved one, death of parents, friends going away, upset at thieves who've stolen things, fired or leaving a job, moving, children growing or going off, physical ailments, or getting old. Resentments play a part in suffering, too. The more unaddressed grudges one carries, the more unpleasant feelings are stashed away. Then we try to bear up under the weight of those suppressed emotions. Often complaints are an indication that the suffering level is high.

Other things that makes us suffer include tolerating what we think is intolerable, replaying memories of abuse, not getting the help we believe we are entitled to, and having unresolved issues from childhood.

The stack grows. A spark ignites. The broken shoelace is too much. What doesn't kill creates a world-class sufferer.

Toward the end of lunch the monk paused, then said, "Let's just call it craving. Either for something or to avoid something. Being stuck in one's rigid opinions or, fighting against the forces of life or refusing to engage in its flow will do it too."

"So, now what?" I asked.

"Well, I'll tell you, but you're not going to like it."

Now quite engaged in this discussion, I said, "We've come this far, lay it on me!"

"You've got to let go of everything. Forgive everyone for everything, even yourself." Then he just looked at me with that quizzical smile, and said, "You get the check!" We hugged and parted.

We'd stayed in touch by phone, but I hadn't seen him for a while until he appeared in my hospital room. At my bedside he said little, just put his hand on my sheet-covered leg. Small talk ensued for a minute or two. With all of the seriousness he could muster he whispered, "Had enough? It's time for you to join up, quit thinking you need something else. Get busy out there. I love you." He turned and walked away.

WHERE WAS SHE IN ALL OF THIS?

Not a surprise that "she" wasn't anywhere to be found in this drama. That's the life of a loner, all right. Male friends showed up, for sure; but nary a girlfriend, ex-spouse, nor sister made their physical presence known. Calls, yes. Hugs and kisses, nope. As usual this was of my own making. After that second divorce in '87 left me with only half a heart, I made a decision: "Don't do that again." That's why they call it "burned" –like not touching a hot stove once you've learned what that's like. As in all distasteful events, whether I liked to face it or not, I had had a part in the failure of the marriage. Her name was Kate and we met while I was working at a treatment center for adolescents. It wasn't love-at-first-sight, but some sparks flew. Finishing-up her Masters Degree in Counseling, tall, slender, short blond hair with a touch of a feisty-attitude, we hit it off. Women who can verbally hold their own always get my attention. Since my first divorce in '77 I wouldn't say I'd been alone, more like serial monogamy. Or one-on-one hanging-out, friends-with-benefits as young people say now; except when either of us got too close, someone always left, usually not on pleasant terms.

So at 40, and she somewhere near that, we decided after a couple of months to get married. The basis for any decision is as good as any other it seemed. There's wisdom in waiting, as she was off having an affair with an old lover within three months. Man that really broke my heart. Again. Wounded, resentful, raging, the bond (love?) was not sufficient to see us through that. We parted. Clearly I did not take time to find out who she was; or I just jumped-in anyhow. That was two years before recovery found me; and one more good reason to sober-up. Life seemed to be one unclear event after another, especially in intimate relationships. Being 'self-propelled', not consulting anyone, took me down. One friend named it' the-broken-picker-syndrome'. But every year or two when heart thought it was healed, ready for another go-at-it, a Ms. Right would show up. Like most every affair, excitement drove the connection until the delusion of happy-ever-after crashed, resulting in more scar tissue. Once the six months' worth of thrill expired and "who-we-really-are" emerged, so did "No, thank you." Either she left or I did. A major part of me always went too. That was the kicker; somehow I got emotionally invested and the breakup hurt like hell, lasting months. For years I limped along emotionally, wanting' her', mostly out of loneliness, but knowing that severe pain always came along. Logically, "Don't go there" became the mantra and primary directive. Like most operating strategies, I didn't invent it. History always plays a part; my life is no different.

Because I was raised in an orthodox Christian home, religious principles guided my life. They cut both ways: keeping the honorable path clear, yet seemingly so strict that the other side of life couldn't be as bad as it was preached about. Like the old *Reefer Madness* movie from the '50's, too much of conventional life became a joke. Ultimately the rigor had to go. My first realization that I couldn't believe all that' they' had taught anymore came with the 1968 Democratic National Convention when Mayor Daly's "pigs" beat the shit out of the hippy protestors. I remember coming home from my part-time job at a grocery store, tired, looking at the TV and feeling so angry and discouraged. It wasn't enough to turn me into an outward rebel, though. The "straight and narrow" life had deep roots in me as I came of age in the '60's.

My secondary education was religion-based, all male, and college prep. Since my family was middle class, I worked summers as well as after school to pay for the tuition. Doctors' and lawyers' kids were my cohorts. Graduation from high school in '64 put me into real-life drama that summer: the Vietnam War had blown our world up. Join up and go to war or not? Friends went to Canada, a couple of them died in Southeast Asia. I opted to go to a Roman Catholic seminary in September of 1965. It seemed the natural next-right thing to do. That lasted for a year and a half. The bubble of

'This-will-make-things-right' burst, there. Organized religion lost its magic. I returned to my family, enrolled in college, 'lapsed' into my own quest for a spiritual connection. Seemingly that chapter of my life was behind me. Right!

Recently I told a friend about this time in the seminary and she said, "Oh, that's what's wrong with you!" But when you're in it, you just can't see it. At age 18, five hundred miles away from home, with no real structure, my attitude was "Good God in heaven, free at last!" And that's how I acted. Three semesters later, with not much more than a C average, it came clear to me that the clerical world was not what it was cracked up to be; at least not for me. The spiritual life is an inside job, not one to be guaranteed through a commitment to "the cloth."

Back home I enrolled at the University of Toledo unsure of a major, but working part-time to pay tuition, staying in my parents' basement (since my bed had been taken by one of the other six), driving a beat-up '51 Chevy, attempting to get an education. And the other students had the nerve to shut down the university in 1966. Wending my way through behavioral sciences, finding fraternity life shallow, scared to death of sex (but longing so for female company), I graduated in December 1969, just about the time of the Tet Offensive.

Fortuitously, I was offered a job as a Juvenile Probation Officer. An exemption from military service came, along with the start of my professional life in Corrections. Living the righteous life had arrived. Here I was, 23 years old, advising parents on how to raise their delinquent kids and talking with juveniles about their problems. The blind leading the blind. The problems must have been the errant children's fault. Drug abuse was just becoming noticeable among youthful offenders. Yes, there was a time when drug abuse was not rampant. I certainly didn't do any of that drug stuff, but alcohol use was fine. My family history and possible genetic set-up began its pernicious walk in my life.

While employed at the Juvenile Court I met the first love of my life, Brenda. She was a secretary working full time to put herself through college, aiming at becoming a teacher. Her lithe beauty aside, there was a noticeable touch of spunkiness that drew me to her. She was thin, with short red hair that was somehow more-bushy on one side. She wore heels that went clickity-clack as she walked the terrazzo floors. I was smitten. We flirted for several months, discovering that we had a lot in common. Then that hot, humid night in July, 1970, we both offered our virginities to the other. We each gladly accepted the gift. Given our backgrounds, of course we "had to marry,' not because of a pregnancy, but because of that cultural "if you have sex you have to get married" injunction. Something happened the following winter while we were planning the wedding. I got scared. Maybe it was the realization that I didn't have to marry the first woman I'd slept with. Over Christmas, at a party, I met the second one, Jeanette. And I married her.

Jeannette was far more-gentle, much more accepting than Brenda. Her willingness to let me be me, without criticism, was magnetic. At 24 there was no way to recognize love. She had grown up in an Irish Catholic home, taught junior high school, and had an older brother and a twin sister, Annette. Both sets of our parents thought we were a good match. We traveled and partied well together. What else was there but to get married, right? We got along OK, our sex life was satisfactory, and we had no major fights. (The first and last fight was when we decided to divorce six years later). But we didn't have any real shared interests or hobbies. From my parents I had learned that commitment equaled suffering, so I was not a fan of the "hard times" mentioned in the marriage vows.

Besides, a year after our wedding we were surrogate parents to delinquent boys in a half-way house we started. A couple of years after that we bought ten acres in Montana, sold our belongings, bought a 4-wheel-drive truck, and headed to Missoula for a summer's camp-out. There, we built a log house, and supported ourselves by working at menial jobs. Mostly we were trying to find meaning in our lives. It was a real adventure. Her love helped me become an adult male. But then my behavior became juvenile. I rewarded her by becoming addicted to substances, being unfaithful, and leaving for six months to "study" in Denver. I was certainly not dedicated to our partnership. She did not deserve any of that; but that's what happened. She was right to leave. God was I sad.

When my big depression descended, it occurred one day after our mutual filing. I ingested every drug I could get my hands on to enable me to sit in that courtroom. On our way out the door, I patted her on the butt as she headed for Alaska. Then I went around the corner, fell to my knees and wept bitterly.

Now, tell me: might this have contributed to an un-partnered lifestyle?

CREATIVE INTELLIGENCE (WIIOT)

Something was watching over me. At a mostly conscious level, I have had a life-long interest in what "Creator" means and my part in this scheme of life. As an adult I am more clear about the process, but the quest to find answers has been confusing. Driven to understand, I knew I was not alone; there are many other "seekers." Teachers tried to point the way, but nobody provided me with an adequate answer. I didn't realize that it was a totally personal job; one that I had to undertake and accomplish myself. Like most of us, I was always looking over-there. My parents (who I've come to see were really angels) provided a context for a spiritual journey. Their families steeped them in Catholicism. They did their best to make "The Path" available to me. Many take the road more traveled—the ready acceptance to religion without questioning. However, there was just too much theology (this-and-that I had to believe) required before I could qualify for a place in heaven; so I went exploring. Trying to make sense of a spiritual path is a lot like Louis Armstrong describing jazz: "If I have to explain it, you won't get it anyway." I was on an odyssey, for sure.

Education seemed the right road; my "angels" had pointed me in that direction. Taking the sometimes tough-love support of my parents ("Go to school or get a job and pay rent!"), I earned a college degree with a major in psychology. Surely understanding, insight and perhaps wisdom would follow. No such luck, in my case. The journey continued with clues egging-me-on. A satisfying connection with the Creator eluded me. Like static on the radio or bad reception, it was just not clear. At times I wondered if "the peace that surpasses all understanding" was really available to me without faith in a redeemer, as the preachers said. Could I really get it?

Someone explained that illusion is the six-foot rabbit I imagine in the corner. Delusion is when I take him a carrot and we walk away discussing how he can get onto late-night talk shows. I was hoping I wasn't delusional.

My spiritual quest was a big question mark. Once I believed that doing all of that religious stuff would get me where I wanted to be—that is, what some call "enlightened." But right after Catholic high school, a stint in a monastery barely satisfied that spiritual thirst. In fact more questions emerged: *"You mean I'm just supposed to accept all of these convoluted dogmas about sin (and the various kinds thereof? Am I supposed to believe the Adam and Eve story? Am I supposed to accept the Bible as completely true, every word of it? I don't think so.)"* Others seem to have found "it," why can't I? ("It" being peace and acceptance amid all of the concepts, abstractions and bullshit about God).

Returning to my home at age 19, my first initiative was to rename God as "Carl." My family laughed, humoring me, thinking to placate this errant one. It only got worse. Instead of going to Sunday Mass I would drive my beat up old Chevy to the banks of the Maumee River, reveling in the Presence there. That feeling was good, but it didn't stay with me more than ten minutes, or a mile and a half past River Road. What would it take to have some kind of lasting "God" impact on my life? Maybe something could relieve the drudgery of daily life. It didn't seem like it had to be that way. Aha! Between alcohol, and the "funny looking home-rolled cigarette," I achieved some relief from the day-to-day business of life. But the problem was that I had to come back to this reality, especially "other people's bullshit." Others seemed to deal with this world better than I. Knowing I wasn't alone, I kept inquiring. Those artificially induced feelings of being carefree were fleeting. The real Presence did not come in a six-pack or "dime-bag" of dope. How ironic that arriving at a place of powerlessness with hands-up in surrender opened me for enough humility to access The Way. And that was only the beginning.

I did not even create the search. My ancestral predecessors have left clues to their search on cave walls, precisely placed monuments, and various markers all over this planet. Anthropologists claim that evidence shows humans have always created and worshipped "something." Early human beings found that "something" in nature.

Humans seem to need an "other" to make sense of life and death. Among our cravings is the drive to explain this life. Some of us possess a strong drive to understand. We need to try to comprehend what this life means, as well as all that happens in it—to come to terms with "the basic philosophical questions." "The mystery" eluded me. Actually I did not know what I did not know about it. I could not be still and just observe; letting life (with its troublesome vagaries) just be. Serenity was momentary. I could not stand to be in the Presence for any extended period of time. There was no distinction between what I could change and what I couldn't.

I now see that the need to know was a manifestation of a need to control. Somehow I had lumped my survival with having a direct say-so in almost everything, thinking that if I had input (or if things went my way), then everything would be OK. There were times, I recall, when I was afraid of air travel because I didn't trust the pilot; or refused to sleep on a cross-country auto trip out of concern that the driver would make a mistake. Selfish, self-centered fear, I was to discover later, was at the root of so much anxiety. When my efforts to be in charge finally failed, when over-or-under-the-counter substances no longer assuaged the pain of living, something had to change, immediately and drastically. Life altered, at last, when I surrendered, then undertook a sober, sincere investigation for that Power Greater Than Myself. That was truly the quest of (for) my life. Through reading literature on contemporary religious/spiritual thinking, sitting in meditation, asking others, and discovering the possibility of a kind and loving Creative Intelligence in charge of the universe, the Presence came over *here* into my life instead of staying out there somewhere.

Once I even asked a mentor about this. His name was Angel, an ex-Louisville gangster. I said, "What's this God's Will thing that I've heard so much about?". He looked at me, grinned and said, "Do you know what the wrong thing to do is?"

"Sure," I said. Mentally I scoffed at the question.

"Then don't do that!"

I thought about that for a moment. "That can't be all of it," I said.

"When you wake up in the morning, ask for guidance, then go help someone."

Simple instructions for a guy who knew The Path had to be complicated. Since that time I've been able to fill in some of the blank spots in his equation; but put simply, he had it right–or when this student was ready, that teacher appeared. Life shifted as I quieted myself and relaxed let-go of manufactured worries and complaints, and focused instead on gifts and blessings. The quest continues today, but without so much angst. Our hands (mine and the Creator's) seem to be on the control stick of my life; it's more like managing the journey. As long as I attend to Who is really in charge, reach out to help others, and perform the rituals for self-maintenance (including things like physical exercise, mental-attitude adjustments and prayer), then I seem to have a better than average shot at being happy, joyous, and free.

By the way, Motorcycle Michael has named the Force "WIIOT," which means "Whatever It Is Out There." That's good enough, today.

GOIN' HOME

Without much hoopla, the day finally came when I left the hospital. What I had been hoping for turned out to be a great change of venue, except my weak, hardly able self was there.

A few days before the big event, I cornered the discharge social worker in her office. Wide-eyed, breathing heavy from dragging my butt there, I tried to convey to her the absolute necessity of my exit, ASAP. One of the nurses had made the mistake of letting slip that the longer one is hospitalized the more the chance of contracting some bug running loose in the facility, like MRSA. That's Methicillin Resistant Staphylococcus Aureus, which is a new strain of infection. I had enough of my own recovery to handle without a volunteer coming aboard for a free ride. "Please let me go home," I begged in a plaintive voice, mimicking a cry. Most social workers are softies at heart, so I was tugging at what I thought was the right string.

Meeting my pleading with a soft understanding tone, she said, "Part of the problem is that wound vacuum attached to your arm. Insurance won't cover your leaving with it, so we have to figure a way for you to go without it.

"Is that all?" Using what I had learned those years in sales, I put my best persuasive foot forward to her. "Would you let me go if I can figure a way to have a nurse change the dressing every other day?"

"Well, I believe that would take care of that situation," she said." But the other concern is that you live in the mountains alone. You seem too weak to take care of yourself right now."

My first wife said I could sell refrigerators to Eskimos, so in that confident "salesman" voice I asked, "What if I stayed with a friend in town?" I was desperate and knew if I was just wheeled out the door, I could handle what I needed, out there.

"Let me talk to your doctor and see if that's satisfactory." Smiling, I retreated backward out her office door expressing my gratitude. Hobbling back down the hallway I reached in my pocket for the prayer beads I'd been carrying. They'd been my companion since '97 when I returned from working in Saudi Arabia. Purchased in Cairo, made of camels' teeth, barely hanging together, they'd served me for nine years. So what if they were designated for Muslims, my conception of the Creator didn't care what beads I used, only that I mumbled incantations. Every time I reached in my pocket they reminded me of my right place–a spiritual entity having a human experience. Over the years, if nothing else, I'd learned how to ask the Infinite Intelligence of the universe for assistance. It helped when I prayed in the spirit of nonattachment to the outcome; except this time I was attached. I really missed my home in the mountains, as it was fall and the colors were changing. Mostly the conifers remain green, but scrub oak, cottonwood by the river, and aspens in the high country put on a show. Besides, my pal Steve had said a few days earlier that I could come stay in his spare room in town for a while.

Patience was called for. I knew leaving was coming. We all have had this happen: some well founded intuition about an event; but waiting is not my strong suit. *"Enough of this hospital, already"* I heard myself think over and over. The background chatter from that mind was on high volume. Putting my exit plan together involved another angel besides Steve, whose offer for refuge was ultimately accepted.

Nettie, a mountain neighbor a couple of miles north, had unexpectedly paid me a visit a couple of weeks earlier in the ICU. She was a registered nurse, and her work was mainly one-on-one with severely handicapped patients. The first week, when I was lying pretty helplessly in that bed, she appeared, bringing Ralph, her paraplegic client, along. Hospital visitations are awkward to begin with. Not knowing Ralph, nor having seen her for several months, pleasantries were all I could muster. The encounter did not last long. What did linger in a mental file was the statement she made as she walked out the door, "Let me know if there's something I can do for you." Now, as I was getting ready to leave, there was.

She was not really the gregarious type, but she knew how to carry on a good conversation once engaged. Her smile was infectious. Over the last few years I'd witnessed her compassion for all creatures, but especially for victims of almost any injustice. Later I found out that her parents were survivors of a Nazi concentration camp and still alive. She was about five feet tall healthy, and no stranger to physical exercise. She reminded me of a woman in a Wagnerian opera, but without the horned hat. She lived spartanly in an old hunting cabin. Her home is quaint, filled with items scattered about from hikes she'd taken or interesting places she'd visited. "Homey" best describes her character, and she had a very easygoing demeanor. We got along well, right off the bat. Still I was surprised when she sauntered into my room with her charge. At her second visit, near the end of my hospitalization, I asked her if she would be willing to change the dressing on the hole in my upper left arm left by the flea bite.

"Of course," she responded eagerly. "We'll have to get some dressing material." In fact, Nettie was my transport out, accompanying me to the hospital pharmacy for supplies that were generously given, on our way out.

The end of September 2006 saw a date established for my exit. Though exuberant, I wondered how I was going to make it; after all, I could barely walk. With winter coming, firewood had to be cut, split and stacked. That took work, which took strength, which took muscle. Six weeks in a hospital bed and a one-to-one tangle with the plague had cost me more than forty pounds, not all of them fat. I lost muscle that I would never get back. If there is a balance in the universe, somebody, somewhere got it.

Dan and Nettie got me to friend Steve's porch where I sat in a round, bowl-shaped bamboo chair curled up with a blanket over me. Deposited there on Labor Day along with bags of goods, my nurse and helpers made me comfortable. While I was sequestered in the hospital, someone brought me a water fountain. A water fountain! On my exit I gave it to brother Dan who appreciated it, I think. Still there were two garbage bags of impedimenta in my little room at Steve's.

For several days in a row I dragged myself from the bed in his spare room to the front porch in a quiet city neighborhood, facing south. Although there was an overhang sheltering my seat, the sun shined on me. My head would fall back, my body go limp as I basked in the warmth, allowing whatever healing there was to permeate my being. It would just take time. Directly across the street were the biggest cottonwood trees I'd ever seen, in the beginning stages of shedding leaves. I sat dazed for hours in quiet reflection, every now and again brought to tears by happenings of the last few months. Reality struck when my caretaker pal said, "Would you like to take a shower"?

"No thanks," I responded slowly. It seemed like too much trouble.

"Let me draw you a bath," he suggested quietly, winking his right eye and heading toward the bathroom before I could answer. That really was what I needed: someone to take over management of the simple things of life. Rarely, it seemed, had I let people do things for me. This encounter with helplessness had brought me that lesson also.

Reinforcements Arrived

Support from friends continued after my release from the hospital. When I finally convinced brother Dan that I could care for myself at home, friends met us there. Mark and Sonja, the "granola type" couple, were at the house when we arrived after a week at Steve's. They had food for me—something I hadn't even thought about. Travelers know the feeling of coming home. Wow, I had made it back! While Sonja warmed the veggie fest, Mark got a pail of warm water and began to scrub my floor. It's a small place, but his gesture and Sonja's moved me to a tear.

We ate quietly. I was struck wordless when Mark asked me what it was like being there. They had recently moved from Arizona, purchased land off-of-the-grid, and built a small straw bale guest house while making plans for a larger one. Three months later when I was getting more mobile I was able to help them lay out their concrete pad for their larger home. Then the next summer I lent a hand with finishing the inside. I gave that payback with joy.

That first week being home was bittersweet. Hobbling twenty feet down the driveway to my truck was the exercise I needed, but I had to rest every time I walked. I caught myself grunting and exhaling loudly after what many would call minimal movement. A caretaker would not have helped me, for I was forced to undertake my own physical therapy just to do usual everyday tasks.

The following Saturday two pickup trucks and four men with chainsaws showed up to cut a winter's worth of firewood for me. Gratitude descended on me, again. It did, however, take me several days of forced rest to recover from that exercise; and I only walked around with them, tossing an occasional log into a truck. The laughter and camaraderie brought a smile that lasted a week, until the CDC lady called.

During the second week back home I received a phone call from a representative of the Centers for Disease Control—or CDC. She said that she would like to interview me for a research project about the plague. "Sure, that's OK with me. If I can be of some help I'll do it." We made an appointment.

When she arrived I was so weak that I was still in my pajamas and robe. Nobody said I had to dress for guests. I did, however, have coffee for her that morning. After we exchanged amenities, she said that some other victims had contracted the plague from house pets. My reply was to ask her what constituted a "pet." To my surprise she said, "They have a name." I smiled. Not trying to be difficult, I told her that the wild animals in the yard are special to me, and I've even named them. The rabbits are Bunny-satva (after Bodhisattva, a Buddhist incarnation); the birds are Bill, Tom, and Kenny. Leftovers from meals go to the coyotes, Sam and Bob, and their families. She was attractive, well dressed, and had a smile that lit-up my morning. She gave it to me in response to my story. I think that she thought that I was kidding. I wasn't.

There was not much more to the conversation, so she politely excused herself. As she was driving away I noticed I had a real interest in a female human being. Survival had replaced that in the Intensive Care Unit. So maybe, just maybe I was making it back to life.

EPILOGUE: THE CORRECTIONS YEARS
A Trail of Tales

Debilitated, as I dragged myself about after hospital discharge, I could barely walk, let alone work for a wage. Four months after I was released from my deathbed, friend Tom talked with me about helping him remodel an old home. With a good crew, I was able to provide tools and direction to complete a beautiful add-on. While on the job I rested every hour just to keep going as work was good physical therapy. The crew knew my situation and understood. This was a small one-bedroom, almost-crumbling adobe built in the 1930's whose plumbing and electrical infrastructure would surely fail any inspection. We did a great job. About the time that ended, I was running out of money. Then I met Parachute Charlie. That moniker landed on him from his days of jumping out of airplanes.

Sadly, one day the life-saving, billowy cloud attached to his back did not fully open, and now he gets around on crutches. Though movement-challenged, one would not know it from his activities, the car he drives, or the education he's achieved. He is licensed as a vocational counselor. About a year after I was discharged from the hospital, I talked with him—but mostly listened to what he had to say. After he asked how I was doing, I relayed my tale of flea-bitten woe. He commiserated, then suggested I contact the New Mexico Division of Vocational Rehabilitation.

Several weeks after my call to them, I found myself seated across the desk from the counselor presenting my story. Gary is well over six feet tall with a smile at least that size. He showed genuine concern for my situation, and asked for a Release of Information so that he could confirm the details of my hospitalization from the records. Two weeks to the day after our first meeting, he called and said that the documents had arrived. With anticipation I hustled myself to the appointment the next day. Barbara, the gal Friday in the spacious office, welcomed me. The office is 30 miles east Albuquerque, and there's something about a rural setting that brings out the more genuine in people. Perhaps it is the lack of pretense. There was no carpeting, no paintings on the wall, and the furnishings were from the early secondhand store period. I felt at home. I had never sought help from a state agency, except the beloved unemployment office. I didn't expect much from this encounter.

As I took a seat across the desk, counselor Gary pulled up my case on the computer, looked at me and said, "You really do need some help, don't you?" Still emotionally raw, I was moved to a tear. Someone actually understood the seriousness of my situation, maybe better than I did. At that point I was still feeling confused, having no idea what I was going to do for work.

I loved building things, but I'd lost so much muscle mass from six weeks on my back that I couldn't even lift a good construction saw. There was no way I could go back into that profession; and I knew it. Gary saw that right away. Being so physically drained, I usually did not have enough energy left to accomplish a task once I arrived at a destination. It was a workout just getting into my truck. Gary asked if there was another occupation for which he could provide training. I was 60, had a few years until retirement, and was broke. Once upon a time I had been a licensed social worker and alcohol counselor. It looked like I was going to be called off of the bench to go back into that game. Noting that as a viable option, he asked, "What would it take to get you back into that field?"

"Probably just applying for a license," I said reluctantly. Six years earlier I had relinquished my professional right to practice because of burnout. I was just plain tired of it. When my licenses expired, I moved into something I'd always wanted to do: building structures. Now, the collision of coincidences was edging me back there to a helping profession. "OK, I'll reapply for my license."

Then Gary observed, "You'll need new glasses, it looks like. How's your hearing?" Truthfully, I'd been saying, "What'd you say?" a lot more lately. Due to a childhood incident, my right ear did not catch sounds as well as the left one. He was quick to offer a hearing test as well as glasses for my next job, whatever it was to be. I got the referrals, thanked him, and headed out the door with a smile.

There was a bulletin board just to the left as I exited. On it were various employment possibilities. One was for the local county jail that also served as a private prison. Since I had some experience in that field, and it was only twenty miles away, I decided to take a leisurely drive checking out that facility. Besides, my job angel had given me a gas card to pay for the search. I'd struck gold. After the trials of the last few years, my luck was changing. On the drive there, however, I realized "luck" was not the right word. Perhaps "grace" was more appropriate. I reveled in it as I drove across the barren flats of the New Mexico desert. Something came over me: a touch of happiness and joy. Strange that it hadn't visited me in a while.

Once in Estancia, I remembered that this is a very different world. Unlike knocking at a neighbor's door, one must be granted admission through the barbed-wire-covered rolling gate via an intercom. By the way, waiting is the game, until the person pushing the OPEN button is good and ready to do so. Welcome to patience. No cell phones, tobacco products, knives, guns or explosives allowed. Now I remembered one of the reasons I did not like these places. The outer gate was just the beginning. Next the metal detector was the portal that awaits all. Metal buttons on my vest set it off, which got a uniformed officers' attention. A-once-over with an electrical wand cleared me. I was hoping they wouldn't make me strip. The next requirement was to empty all pockets and send the contents through a security pass-through for review. After I got the thumbs-up from behind the bulletproof glass, I was granted entry.

The officer in charge motioned me to sit while he made a call to Human Resources. Shortly, a young lady came down a corridor, smiling. When I inquired about job openings, she said that there was only one available: Alcohol Counselor. Well, how about that? Being in the flow of positive circumstances elated me. Finally I felt like I was truly in the 'zone'. Since I'd had the license previously, it did not seem a large hurdle to obtain it again. However I soon leaned that one other critical piece of information I hadn't seen in forty year was required: a copy of my high school diploma. High school diploma!!?? Not since 1964 when it was granted had I seen hide-nor-hair of it. Leaving the facility, I made a mental checklist of tasks to complete. Would my old secondary institution even have records back that far? Did those four years only exist in my memory?

Yes, I really *did* graduate–the record did exist–and within thirty days I was employed at the County jail/private prison, new glasses on board, hearing aids ordered. A familiar if not uncomfortable world was re-opening. But it wasn't your everyday workplace.

Some nerve is needed to survive in a prison, inmate or employee. Having walked main corridors before, I was not initially shocked as I had been the first time. That was in Santa Fe right after the 1980 riot that left thirty-three dead. Since the Corrections Training department I worked for at the time had loaned the New Mexico State Police a video camera to first film the carnage, I was invited on a "tour" shortly after that event. I was aghast at the blood. To see a supposedly secure building look like a war zone deeply troubled me; and to visit the place where not a month before men had brutally taken other lives and lost their own, hurt my soul.

Main hallways in lockups limit access in and out. That's the first way security is managed. Even though experience can minimize fear, there's still a bit of an inner jolt when that large rolling steel gate clunks shut. Suddenly you're in there...with them. The sound has finality to it, along with the vision of "locked-in." Looking around at inmates strolling next to me was another awakening. Thieves, rapists, even murders seem to have heightened sense when incarcerated, always looking for prey. I was being eyeballed. Experience has taught me that much. They can smell fear. I tried not to give off the odor. There's no deodorant for that. Trying to look cool seemed the best course of action, as well as remaining close to uniformed officers. A lot of good that would really do, since they carry no weapons. It's the "cop in their mind' as one official told me. Most men doing long sentences know the score: they just do their time, staying out of trouble as much as possible. But all inmates have a scam: some do art on envelopes or on others' bodies (tattoos, which are illegal), or ink on handkerchiefs. Items are traded; barter is one of the games. To survive one must know the rules. Breaking them has penalties, most of which are swift and harsh. Injunctions are:

1. Get in with a group you think you can trust; but there's a price for that, too.
2. Get a tattoo–the more the better.
3. Fight when you must to prove that you can't be had.
4. If you submit, be prepared to go all the way–you'll end up someone's "bitch."
5. Always keep your eyes open–someone wants something from you.
6. If you give away something, get something of more value in return.
7. Never snitch–you will ultimately suffer.
8. Know who's really in-charge; and it's usually not who you think it is.

Failure to do these has basically two consequences–well, only one: you get physically hurt. Either you are thrown out of the group, left alone as prey, or dead.

This was the world I'd entered. Keeping myself separate from that disorder meant high vigilance. Pay attention, Michael, or become prey. That was drummed in during the initial induction conference after I was hired. Getting acclimated in this particular facility involved a week's worth of training about security as well as policies and procedures. In truth, it was boring. But in between sessions my boss in the Education department wanted me there. Located apart from the main facility, there were three locked doors to get "buzzed through."

I was assigned as the Substance Abuse Education Counselor, and my job was to present classes about drug and alcohol abuse. There wasn't much education to be given; the students thought they knew more than the instructor. What was really missing for them were awakenings to the consequences with motivation to change. They had a hard time connecting their drug use to incarceration. Duh! That was my job as I saw it, plus record keeping as my boss saw it. Tracking results, if only who attended and what assignments were turned in, was a big part of the job. Whether anyone changed their lives or decided never to return to prison, that was a bonus.

Regarding paperwork, I had been baptized by fire in this area by a boss thirty years earlier, and not too gently, either. At a treatment center, a wise administrator got in my face about my documenting insufficiencies. Two days before payday he called me into his office and said, "Here in my left hand are charts that must be completed. In my right hand is your paycheck. Do we understand each other?" We did. Needless to say I got the lesson, and the paycheck. That first job in a substance abuse treatment center taught me so much, as well as launching me on a career, not to mention providing me another step into personal recovery. There's a pattern to success.

It's about sticking with what one does–well. Talk to any long-timer in any field. No doubt one will hear of years of practice.

I didn't have all of my confidence back yet. Thankfully the Internet provided assistance with lesson plans. I reviewed old files, prepared a flyer to attract students, and within three weeks held the first class. Seven brave souls showed up. Roll taken, syllabus distributed, it was time for introductions. Another rule "inside" is "Don't talk (or give away information) unless your life depends on it–then lie." Knowing the operating conditions helped. Starting by telling about myself might break some of the ice. Sometimes personal disclosure will open others. It didn't. As each man stated his name, a mini question and answer session followed, mostly low-threat, "safe" information. Home town? Married? Kids? Time "down" (slang for incarceration period)" Knowledge of substance abuse? With the last question I hoped that someone would say that they had a problem in this area. Once one domino fell, the others would. It did. As an instructor I made an effort to be "just another guy." That worked, too. Then one of the more assertive students asked, "What are you doing in this place? You're a smart guy. You don't need to be in here like us."

That was the opening I was waiting for. With some humility (after all, the classroom door was closed and I was within striking distance of junkies, weightlifters, as well as assaulters), I opened up. Revealing the story of my life, particularly as it related to substance abuse counseling-education, was not difficult. Leveling the playing field was what I was after, for as a rule, staff members have hardly any credibility in institutions. I was not trying to be their friends, but it was a strategy to get trust and openness going. It worked. It was also potentially lethal. Giving the "enemy" ammunition isn't the wisest move; but I did not see them as the enemy, as others in the facility did. I was not Security (walking around with handcuffs on my belt) I was in the Education department. There were moments of fear, when I was jammed shoulder-to-shoulder with inmates in a crowded hallway in the separate building that housed classrooms. Help, in an emergency, was three locked gates away, five minutes, anyhow. That was part of the job. Staying on my side of the imaginary relationship fence was crucial. Getting too friendly is dangerous. It was a thin line...reaching out to help another, but not being grabbed by the other reaching back.

As is usual in any normal distribution, there were two men in the group who responded to the verbal bait by sharing information about themselves, two who were neutral, and two who sat scowling. Then there was the guy who sat apart from the group, even after being invited to the table. Clearly he was playing by his own rules. Probably 5 foot 9 inches, stocky like a football player who played tackle, well tattooed, with a shaved head, a blank stare, and a very reserved smile. This guy knew and played well the "con game." He wasn't about to give anything, questioned everything, and volunteered nothing. Like the others, Franko was there for the "good time," reduced sentence for successfully completing an educational program. At least the others showed some willingness. There was only one way to get him to participate: he had to be "one-up-ed," but not invalidated in front of the others. Speaking up was not his problem. He was articulate, once he spoke. At some level he was aiming for top dog position in my classroom. Clearly he wanted me to take him on; but "putting him down" would have cost me. Thankfully I'd bantered with enough guys to know the game. So, we went at it in the second session. After introductions again, and questions about unfinished homework, we began verbal sparring:

"So, you did the homework. Anything you realized from it?" I asked.

"Not much. I've been through this so many times," was his reply.

"I have a suggestion if you'd like it."

"What's that?" he said, looking directly at me, trying to camouflage a sneer.

"I don't know if you really want to change your life. But if you do, you might want to do something else rather than the same-old-same-old." He nodded, shifted his head a bit to the right, stuck out his lower lip in acknowledgement. It was a Scarface sort of response. The point had been made and taken. Score one for the Teach.

Then here came the return salvo. "Something's gotta be different. This gets real old and so am I. Don't get me wrong–I can hold up my end of anything. But there's stuff I wanna do out there. I'm here on a bogus parole violation, so I'm waitin' til it gets cleared up."

"Tell me how anything's got a chance to be different if you keep doin' the same old stuff? That's the real definition of insanity: doing the same thing hoping it'll all be different, no? I'd be willing to bet that the same old cast of characters keep doing the stuff you've always done in the places you always hang out at."

"You're right about that," he admitted. "So you think you can teach me something new about dope and the streets?"

M: "Probably not. But you can get out of your old thinking and look at yourself from another angle. Einstein said. 'The significant problems we face cannot be solved at the level of thinking we were at when we created them.' You gotta go at it differently. Now I know something about that."

Silence.

"Give me an example, will you?

"Sure. I'll bet that you believe it is somebody else or something else that has always gotten you in trouble. What if you had something to do with it. Like all of it?"

"I'm not sure that's true. These other guys got me hooked on dope, then I followed them into crime, then somebody snitched me off, then this guy attacked me, then I got locked up. All that's not my fault."

"You don't strike me as a victim, dude. So who did all of this happen to? And who was there in all of the bullshit that happened to you? My guess would be you...that you had something to do with all that. Who went along into dope? Who went along on the crime sprees? Who set himself up to be snitched off? Not me. Without being too personal, I'd say it was the guy in the chair across from me. Brother, the only way I can see to get any clarity, and a new way to look at it, is for you to own up to your part in your life. Like it or no! Do it or don't. Your life."

"Man, you don't pull no punches, do you? I'll have to think about this. It puts a whole new meaning on all of the bullshit in my life. I think I'd rather go on blaming somebody else. It looks easier. Thanks anyway, doc."

"You're welcome. Remember that you're the one who wants things to change. Ain't nobody going to wave a magic wand to fix things. The bad news is YOU gotta do it. Class dismissed."

No more classes were scheduled that week due to a lockdown of all inmates and then the weekend. On Monday morning as I was walking in the crowded corridor with wall-to-wall orange suits, a hand grabbed my right arm, tightly, pulling me to the wall. It was Franco.

" Look man, you are right on about everything you said, but I can't open up in there with those other guys. Can I talk to you in private about this after class?"

"Sure," I said. "But I want something from you–I want you to participate with the others. You know, like answer some questions when I ask. They respect you, and I need some help here."

"You got a deal, man."

And he kept his word. That class went well, homework got done, participants started participating, there were no incidents right to the end. During the last of the twelve-week sessions I was told that the State of New Mexico inmates were to be moved out of this private prison to another. Only Federal and Immigration offenders were to remain. The bad news was that those Federal inmates did not qualify for education classes. The department was to be disbanded. In an address to the staff, the warden assured almost all of those present that their jobs would continue, except a few. I was in the select group whose heads rolled, a couple of hours west.

Shortly thereafter I was called to the Chief's office for a chat. He told me that I was to be furloughed unless I chose to move 150 miles west to the women's prison operated by the same private company. There was an opening for a counselor in the substance abuse program. Coincidental cards played again, as my profane spiritual teacher, the monk, worked in that facility. He was living in a one-bedroom apartment. My body has never been averse to a sofa in a strange town, when needed. Off I went the next week, and it was only 100 miles from my home. Four nights a week we hung out together, sometimes meditating, more often munching our way through a football game; and I don't even like sports. Golf is really his thing, so I was strongly invited to participate–friends do that to each other. The workweek was spent in that lockup of insane progesterone, some evenings at the driving range.

There's a real difference between women's and men's prisons– Duh! But there are some things that are recognizable in both. Put people with a defiant disorder in a place of restricted freedom and watch what happens. This does not breed happy campers. As a matter of fact, residents better learn "use-or be used." As in any community there are operating conditions, but in correctional facilities these are based on survival. I moved from a men's facility where power and fear were injunctions, to a women's where subtle manipulation was in effect. Now, that was educational, if not downright dangerous. The behaviors were different, of course, and less obvious.

Being a man, a lot more attention came my way: blinking eyes implied availability and coyness. I just had a similar but different target painted on me. Exploit or be exploited. But I slid into getting along. Since I grew up with four sisters and was managed by an assertive mom, women's ways are familiar. But being hard-wired male, all of the attention occurred like flattery, especially coming from younger females to an older male. In almost any other context it would have felt great; it only put me on alert. The facility-specific training about sexual assault perpetrated by a staff member being a felony, was taken seriously. No one knew that the education director in this facility would be evicted for just such an offense in a few months. Having made my boundary clear to several of the students, word spread that I was actually "safe" to talk to. Interactions got easier as well as more honest when the "flirting cloud" lifted.

Several staff members had coached me about boundaries with the women. One was Jerry, a licensed therapist in the psychology department. Lunches were highlights of the day when we would exchange witticisms, puns and insights. After a couple of months he took a job back in Albuquerque, where he lived. Shortly after his departure, he called me with an invitation to come to work with him. Three days later I was sitting in an interview at the Metropolitan Detention Center in Bernalillo County, located out on the mesa west of Albuquerque.

More money and a site fifty miles closer to home drew me to the interview. Dr. U. was the head psychiatrist in the Psych Services Department. In all of my years sitting with potential employers, I have never spent such an inspiring time. For my part I'd become much more honest, and could distinguish bullshit from truth with skill. After the opening pleasantries I asked about the job, though I'd seen the written description. His South American accent belied his profound understanding of the English language. Articulate without resorting to "shrink" language, he told me about interviewing inmates who were requesting psychoactive medication for mental disorders. Each sentence communicated compassion. I was stunned. Then I found myself asking a strange question, "Have you ever been moved to tears in an interaction?"

He looked at me with a serious expression, but also a hint of a smile he said, "Of course." That commenced a most amazing moment of pregnant silence; one I'd never had previously. In that quiet between us we communicated more than any lengthy questionnaire or standardized test. Time stood still. We truly beheld each other.

The third person sitting with us couldn't take the intensity, so she said something like, "Well, we have that clear." That broke the moment, but not the bond. Next she asked if I'd like to take an application. I responded, "Actually I do not like filling those out, unless I'm going to get the job."

She looked at Doctor U. "What do you think?"

"Yes, offer it to Michael" was directed at both of us. That was it. A month later, after obtaining a security clearance, I started the new job. What a team that man assembled! From a large room full of eighteen cubicles, we did amazing diagnostic and intervention work. None of us missed the weekly staff meetings. With anecdotes full of wisdom he drew out the best in each professional, even during conflict. Within six months we became co-creators on a mission, to the point where he would entertain unusual questions of a personal nature. Once when alone he seemed particularly quiet. I asked him if something was troubling him. He motioned me into his office and we sat down. While he settled into his favorite rocking chair, he took off his glasses, positioned himself to see me, much like he had during our first meeting. He said, "This is the anniversary of my daughter's death four years ago." A couple of tears came to his eyes. Quiet, again. I was, too. My eyes could not contain their moisture, either. That was an eternal five minutes.

"I'm sad that happened," I said. That seemed inadequate, but it was the best I could do.

"Yes," he said. "Is there anything that I can do for you?"

"You are doing it, now," he said in a slow exhale. Moments later we stood at the same time, and embraced. It reminded me of the last time I had hugged my father. We held each other a bit longer than usual. "Thank you," he said.

"Yes, thank you, also" was all I could say. We parted.

Almost exactly two years from my first day of work, after a busy Friday the feisty supervisor, Mary, called me into her office. Ours was a great relationship, full of humor, but with well acknowledged mutual boundaries. With sadness in her voice, she said, "Today is your last day. Our new contract contains requirements for licensure, which you do not have. You must clear out your desk, return your badge, and leave."

Of course I was shocked. "Oh, that's pretty simple, isn't it? Has my work been less than satisfying?"

"Not at all. You are one of our best. I've never seen anyone relate to inmates like you do. And they really listen to you. It's the corporate office. Here is a letter and three months of compensation, plus you can get unemployment. I'm really sorry about this." In a fog, I hugged her, left her office and shuffled to my good friend David's' desk. When I told him what had happened, his expression told me he was sad and angry. With his help we emptied my desk, said our farewells, then I headed for the only exit from the jail. It was one of those moments of accepting an unacceptable reality. It was hard to believe that I would not be back on Monday.

When I got to my car I called Keith, my mentor. He said, "I don't know whether to say I'm sorry or congratulations."

"Probably both are right," I said.

Attacked!

In all my years working in Corrections–prisons as well as jails–I've never been physically hurt...until yesterday, June 6, 2013. Even some proficiency at martial arts did not prepare me for being blindsided. One minute I was talking, the next I was on the floor cupping my hand to my chin, bleeding into it. A set of broken dentures came out of my mouth, floating in that palm-full of sanguineous mess. Eyeglasses were gone, probably lying on the floor.

"What happened? I think I just got hit! Where the hell did that come from? These guys are chained-up. Whoa, those CO's (Correctional Officers) are all over that guy. I think I'm all right. Can I stand? Yep. Oh, thanks for the hand up. Man, my mouth hurts. There's the head nurse helping me walk. Yes, I can follow your finger left to right. I have a busted upper lip? Please get me out of here..."

Certainly I'm not the only guy to whom this has happened: cold-cocked, knocked down with one punch. What makes this different? It occurred in a group counseling room, in a jail with high-risk inmates who have a history of violence. Oh, also all seven men were in handcuffs, leg cuffs with a short chain running between the two in front of them. On top of this, each was shackled to the wall. One would imagine this was a safe situation. Think again, Mr. Assume All Is Well! Accidents seem to go that way, don't they; and in a blink of an eye, as well? But there it is. The next immediate thing one was going to do, is just not going to happen. It's best to have a backup plan in one's hip pocket, including HELP. That includes friends. Life is very, very unpredictable.

At the time of the assault I didn't immediately feel serious pain. Correctional Officers sitting right outside of the door pounced on the offender in a heartbeat. "Staff down" came over loudspeakers while an ear-piercing beep shot through the facility via air horns located everywhere. Quickly, thirty or more uniformed officers showed up. The whole facility was immediately locked down– 2,500 incarcerated souls were placed back in their cells. The things we learn, mostly from TV shows, about violence in jails against almost anyone, are basically true. Before I knew it (of course I was in shock so time stopped, dead), Maggie, the friendly charge nurse, was helping me to my feet. Every locked facility has a medical team located inside: a mini-hospital... Emergency Room and all. They handle sick calls, do diabetes tracking, administer various tests (including those for pregnancy), tuberculosis exams for all inmates, as well as treatments for every real and supposed complaint. These are seasoned professionals who possess major amounts of patience. Walking a thin line between compassion about a situation and the need to say NO when a subtle request for medication requires a tactful response, those medical folks have street smarts.

Since most residents are in various stages of detoxification from substances, nursing staff and physicians are busy 24/7. Emergencies in the cellblocks require immediate intervention. There is a modified golf cart complete with medical equipment driven by EMTs to the emergencies. Maggie took my arm to assist me to the cart.

How are you feeling?" she asked.

Since I was OK enough and we were good buddies, I responded, "I'm mostly fine. By the way, could you take me home tonight?"

She laughed and turned to the small crowd, "He's all right, being rude, as usual."

After my short ride back to nursing central, one of the doctors pronounced me well enough to go to an outside ER. My wounded pride rode along, so did embarrassment. I did not like being the center of attention...my five minutes of fame was attained at age seven in Toledo, Ohio when I was on some hokey kids' show. Being the victim of an assault, having several hundred people discuss the event–this was not what I would have created. Life happens! We all want life to go our way. That's human. My plan for the next twelve weeks did not include this; that's for sure. It looked more like: keep working, save money, help as I could, then retire again at the end of the summer. This particular early June afternoon had me headed to the Occupational Medical Facility for an exam, accompanied by my boss, bloody towel held to my mouth. After a piss-test to determine that I was not intoxicatingly responsible for the event, I was seen by the Physician's Assistant. Salt-and-pepper gray haired, fit, 5 feet 10 or so, he looked like a young version of Tom Sellick. "At least your jaw is not broken, nor do you have a concussion–you were really pretty lucky, pal," he said. "Sorry this happened. You'll be healed-up in a week or two; maybe have a black-eye, though. You can go back to work tomorrow."

What? You gotta be kidding! Here was a professional sitting across the table from a patient who had no lower teeth, a swollen right cheek and busted lip. This did not seem like an appropriate conclusion. If I went back in that jail, sat across from an inmate, no doubt the first question would be, "What happened to you?" Curtly I would respond: "Accident." Probably that would only precipitate more inquiry. All in all, that wouldn't seem to contribute to the interaction where the focus was on the patient's reason for incarceration, not my black-eye.

The real question should be, "What are you doing in this jail, again?" Or, "Have you had enough of this (bullshit) yet?" Inevitably, the answer would come, "Hell, yes!" Next I'd have to ask, "How do you know?" An interesting dialogue usually ensues with the blame almost-always falling on "chemical dependency." Invariably, incarceration followed–it almost always does. At least this is an attribution the inmate can pin it on, possibly verbalizing it for the first time. For most in this facility this is true. Drug abuse is endemic there.

However, infrequently there is a less identifiable driver: a mental disorder (not that a substance-abuse disorder is not enough). In the verbal interplay, what gets revealed before very long is: physical abuse, pain, suffering or craving have perniciously led to over-or-under-the-counter medication. Legal problems and the lockup follow...a predictable pattern. For some, though, serious mental illness may have been congenital or lying in wait. Perhaps even the result of too much of a difficult life. Obviously not everyone learns how to deal with disappointments, discouragements, or the "slings and arrows of outrageous fortune" with aplomb.

The fellow who clobbered me that day is really, really mentally ill: schizophrenic for sure, with other sidebars of craziness. During the counseling group I was leading, where the attack occurred, I saw him laughing to himself several times. No doubt telling himself jokes he'd never heard before. Inner voices will do that to one, I'm told. On the other hand, I was paying attention to something other than the tightness of his handcuffs. Attempting to be a good listener, as well as facilitator of conversation, I was otherwise engaged, until...down-for-the-count. Once back on my feet in recovery, bodily and mental reactions intruded on me.

Returning to some semblance of normal after an assault is new–this hasn't happened in fifty years. The last one was long ago, but vividly remembered. In high school Richard McNutt, the neighborhood bully, used to drive his hotrod full speed down our street in the 60's. Being a sort of vigilante, my mom called the police because lots of young kids played in the two-lane road. He got back at her by sucker-punching me in front of the burger stand around the corner from the grocery store where I worked after school. That was embarrassing, too. Fighting had never been part of my world. My dad grew up scrapping with his four younger brothers as well as others on the south side of Toledo. Plus he was a WW II veteran. Our family was Christian and unspoken pacifists. My body healed then. It will now. This mind is not as resilient. Of course, shock got me now, like then. Fifteen minutes after the incident in Cellblock 6, I was telling the Chief psychiatrist that the patient was a very sick guy who was going to hit somebody. My face got in his way. Lucky me...understanding did not mitigate the shock. And I didn't even know I was in that state.

At the ER where I was taken, Pam, my friend the nurse, met me, bringing her compassionate indignation along. She knew all of the right questions to ask. After the once-over by the physician's assistant, she took me home. I was noticeably quiet, even to myself. A good night's sleep followed, not induced by medication, and I was not restless. However, the next day a strange unexpected thought came to me out of nowhere: *I have never really lived up to my father's expectations.* Then tears were rolling down my cheeks. "What's this?" that mind asked. It chattered about inadequacy and insufficiency, and my crying became deeper. Then I stopped crying, wiped my eyes, and took a deep breath. I started fretting about retrieving my car, which had been left at the facility. After that: "How do I get new glasses? What about the broken dentures? Where's the aspirin for this headache? Now what?"

Later on, that first day after the attack, I made a phone call to the Workers Compensation office and was put on hold for an extended time. Without warning I got really angry. Cursing and swearing at the phone didn't help...nothing did. "What the hell are you so pissed-off at?" came the question from the same unknown place the last one did. Later that day I made my way home, dealing with a series of drivers who were in the same emotional place that I was: impatience laced with an edge of rage. Fingers flew, brake lights warned, yelling was the communication form, but no weapons. Friend Pam called inviting me to her home. Thankfully I made it. When I was safely at her kitchen table, Pam asked how I was doing.

Like a volcano, venom spewed forth. A lava flow of complaint upon complaint landed on the table. Each one generated another wave of emotion with a higher volume. Finally I couldn't deal with that anymore, and said, "I gotta stop this."

"OK," was her response. Then I quit speaking. Sitting there while we just looked at each other, I grew calm. Her loving eyeball-to-eyeball gaze ameliorated the torrent. Ten minutes must have passed.

Then in a soft tone of voice I said, "This is not me. What's going on?"

Taking my hand, looking right through me she almost whispered:"You were brutally attacked yesterday, remember?"

Demurely I replied, "Oh, right. That's it. That got to me, didn't it?"

In her sweet way, she screwed up her face, crinkled her nose, cocked her head sideways and spouted, "Duh! You need to talk to a professional, pronto!"

The next day I made an appointment to see my primary care physician. As luck and summertime would have it, he was off on vacation. Melissa, his Physician's Assistant, sympathetically listened to my story. I found myself in tears. Handing me a tissue, she noted from the medical record, " You were here eighteen months ago telling the doctor that you felt suicidal. You look depressed to me." For once, and finally, it was that obvious. The lid had gotten blown off of the seething cauldron of resignation and denial, which I thought I had managed for the last fifty-plus years. There it was, right in front of me. This particular characteristic had been kept under wraps for a long, long time. "Yes, sir, it's been hangin' around since I was a kid" came the finally admitting inside voice.

"You probably need some medication to get you stabilized and through this," Melissa said. "Also it would be good for you to talk to a professional. I'll get you a referral." Her kind but firm admonitions got to me. For once my hands went in the air (proverbially, in surrender). That's a tough one for some people, especially of the male variety. It takes steps to do it right. First, I had to let go of an outcome to which I had an attachment ("Managing my own depression, thank you"). Next I had to trust another ("She's right about this thing being out of control."). Finally I put up the white flag.

I had a bit of a "hang dog" attitude and I was disappointed that the situation had come to this. But at the same time a part of me knew it was time to deal with it. Sheepishly I told her, "I thought I could handle this on my own. It doesn't come up very often; but it's always over there, just waiting. "

Doing something different at this point was crucial. Sayings kept coming at me: "Enough is too much", "When you reach the end of your rope, tie a knot and hang on"; "When life gives you lemons, make lemonade." Frankly, I'd had enough of trying to make a tasty beverage out of the fruits I'd been given.

These have to be the simple essential elements that bring about change: get a bellyful, then be willing to try a new thing! After of course, a major event causing an eye-opening, head snapping, "What the hell just happened?" If this were the first emotional ass-kickin' it would be more traumatic. But this was not the first.

Seven years earlier the Bubonic Plague got my attention. Do the lessons ever stop coming? Finally I got to a psychiatrist.

It was strange to find myself in this phenomenological place. Especially to be sitting on the other side of an interview with a psychiatrist. The table had turned.

Maybe, just maybe, from a perspective one might call unconventional, I was coming to a Real-I-zation: Perhaps that crazy guy did me a favor...certainly not anticipated, but here nonetheless. Without this experience, life would have continued as it was–depression well managed (almost), plodding onward through the fog of life. Some things are hard to deny, especially when right in one's face, like a fist.

There's a line from the movie *Tombstone*, when Doc Holliday talks about Wyatt Earp's pending shootout with the cowboys. Someone asks about it, and Doc dubs it a "Reckonin'."

At 66 here it is: Life is Life, I reckon.

BUDDHA IN CHAINS

It's the last place you'd expect to find an honest-to-God real connection to spirituality. Twice a week at one of the largest county jails in the country, there's a therapy group for people in Administrative Segregation. Informally it's known as "the hole." These inmates are locked alone in a 5- foot by 10-foot cell for 23 hours a day, let out by themselves for 30 minutes on the morning and afternoon shifts. With no radio, TV or computer, maybe some reading material and lots of noisy thugs for company, it's not a nice place. Violent residents get this treatment. By the way, when they are brought to the group counseling room, it is in shackles and handcuffs, leg irons with a chain between the two, then anchored to the concrete wall. Lock somebody up like this and see how much "personal growth" they want to engage in.

Not unlike the old cartoon of a hairy troll chained to a dungeon wall wondering where the toilet paper is, therapeutic issues are like the wipes just out of reach. Mental health is not front-and-center on their agenda. Initially I brought them brewed coffee and cookies as a bribe. They knew it; and I agreed when they pointed it out. My request, or thinly veiled demand, was for interesting conversation. They agreed to this. But mostly, complaints were the order of the day:

"Nobody wants to help me" (means "That damned caseworker hasn't dealt with my request")

"Food is bad" (means "more bologna on stale white bread doesn't cut it")

"Not enough time out of my cell" (means "How's somebody supposed to get a shower and make calls in 30 minutes?")

"I can't contact my family" (means "I know she's seeing somebody else")

"I can't sleep in this place" (means "If that guy two cells down doesn't shut up, I'll do it for him")

"The meds aren't working" (means "I need more drugs")

Then finally:

"This is it, I'm never coming to jail, again" (means "Damn, I said it before, I just don't know how to do it")

In the group, once the suffering angels have had a cup of coffee with a cookie, the chatter shifts. Oh... it's nearly impossible to drink with one hand while eating with the other. The chain between the shackles won't allow it. Dunking won't work; neither will crossing one's legs. Standing will, except the chain to the wall won't allow more than a shuffle step. That's control, all right.

As the meeting progressed, each fellow added a personal ingredient to the conversational stew. Of course, jailhouse "smack" (the one-up chatter) had to be managed so it wouldn't escalate to a screaming match, or worse. One inmate, however, sat quietly in the corner. His name was Raoul. He was in his thirties, brown-skinned, well built, and had a teardrop tattooed just below and to the side of his right eye. That teardrop seemed to reflect his mood, and I found out that it did. As the conversation on "change" evolved, he came to. His catatonic state broke when someone spoke the phrase "wake up."

"That's it! That's what's going on. I've been like in shock since they mace-ed me in that cell a couple of weeks ago. That's not all: beanbags from a shotgun, then the damned dog tore up my arm. Before that, I'd had enough of this bullshit and wasn't going to move or do a damned 'nother thing. It took six of those cops to take me down. I still hurt. But, you know what? I just snapped. That's what it took, I guess. It's been two weeks that I've been sitting, bruised up pretty bad. Stuff has been going through my mind about how I've lived."

"Snapped" is street jargon for an enlightenment experience. It's not uncommon for folks whom one might label anti-social to be aware of something that might cause a major shift in their lives. More than once, all of us have imagined a better life. Some think it is magic: lights and mirrors to get to a good life.

A normal life with freedom seems out of the grasp of those caught in the very vicious claws of the corrections system. Once in, it's hard to get out. That black hole has a real suck. "It" (the system) and "they" (the cops) are always waiting, pursuing a person, dogging/hounding a felon for re-arrest, re-incarceration, return to prison, politely called recidivism. That defiant disorder is alive and well. Changing one's life is hard. Being locked up doesn't make it any easier. But it can happen.

Often a trauma has to occur, if one is lucky enough. A really significant reason has to show up before another way can become important enough. Sometimes an accident or other life-threatening event can precipitate a reconstruction of how one is living. For normal folks, ongoing life experiences may be substantial drivers needed to bring about change. Natural processes like graduation, marriage, birth of children, or death can do it. But for someone used to jail, it takes a bit more.

Being locked up is a minor annoyance for those who don't mind it. Actually like life, once the rules are learned, jail's just another place. Many become skilled at the game. In fact, it doesn't take very long to learn the "incarceration tango." Survival and street skills prevail: bully, threaten, get one up or over on another person, certainly "get away with," avoid responsibility, and 'get-high' when possible. When one who is steeped in crime decides to stop while in jail, something seems amiss. That was Raoul.

Not unlike Prince Siddhartha, who found it impossible to continue the life he was living, the man in the corner just stopped. His quiet contemplation surprised even himself. When a language for his experience was made available, he embraced the words. Up to that moment when he could finally make sense of the dilemma, he had been confused, mostly fearful. That's an uneasy admission for a gangster; yet he said it in front of others in the group. This can happen with an enlightenment event: willingness to admit to the truth from which one has been hiding. Because someone doesn't know is not enough reason anymore not to try. In this state, life seems to stop, as the person begins to take stock of his situation. Confusion is certainly present, as re-examination reveals that past patterns will no longer serve. After a time of regret, the searcher struggles to find a recipe for a new life. But the combination of anxiety and anticipation can be a real stopper. Creating a newer, better-adapted life is scary, as new things have to be tried which might have previously been avoided. New people, new places, different thoughts, possible failures occur.

In the group Raoul struggled to say, "I've spent the last week or two thinking about my past—what a mess I've made. People got hurt really bad. My wife and kids are like strangers—stuff happened that I shouldn't have done. I was bad."

Regret combined with shame is powerful, probably appropriate for past actions. Most humans do this. But that doesn't really make anything better—just creates suffering of a different kind. He was open and listening, so I said,

"Dude, you gotta do something different."

Eric jumped in uninvited, "Yeah, aliens don't hang onto shit—they let it go". Clearly psychotic, a regular attendee, he made no bones about being from another planet. Yet what he said applied.

And Raoul heard it, clearly. He came back with, "That's it, for sure. But how do I do that? My whole life's been about crime, from the time I was a kid. The low life has been my life. Regular work, regular people, regular things—man, I don't think I can do that straight life."

Again Eric threw in his sincere two cents worth: "Aliens don't worry either. It's not in their nature. They do what's in front of them. That's all. Especially they don't hurt people. We practice L.G. You could always hop on a ship and try a new life out there."

"What's L.G.?" Raoul asked.

"It's Letting Go!"

Shaking his head and smiling, Raoul responded, "Eric, you're nuts about this space stuff. But I wish I could do that—just let go and be another person. How do I do that on this planet?"

The room was still. Everyone was waiting for my answer. Sucking in a very deep breath for courage, I quietly said, "Making a different and better way for yourself is possible; not easy, but do-able. You gotta start here, now, in those chains. Right in this breath you are an altered person in that High Risk Inmate jumpsuit. Your only problem is living the new you, one step at a time. There is one other small thing for you to consider. You just maybe, might want to consider really growing up—you ain't no kid anymore. There's a time in a man's life when he consciously decides to be responsible. Most guys put it off as long as they can. Some never get it. Now you've got a shot at it."

"You mean I can make up a life I want to live? What should I do?"

Not trying to be a smart ass, I smiled wryly and said, "Welcome to your real life."

People make the leap from victim of their own lives to accomplishing great things, like staying out of jail. This is the real work in life: owning up to how one has lived, deciding on a different kind of life, then living it. Help is usually required. It can be found. He nodded his head in agreement.

Kenton

"You sure are an asshole, aren't you?" Kenton chided me with a tone not altogether unfriendly. There was the hint of a smile on his face.

"Yes sir, I'm just like you," I shot back quickly without a heartbeat between the question and the response. His smile told me that it had been well received. "Now that we've got that clear, what's next?"

These verbal pot shots were exchanged in an interview room in the largest jail in New Mexico between a psychological counselor (me) and an inmate requesting therapy for his thoughts of suicide. There's an art to determining who has an honest-to-goodness real mental disorder requiring medication, from those detoxing in real or imagined pain. Frankly, I was tired of the same old drug-withdrawal bullshit from convicts who wanted pharmaceutical assistance to relieve the pain of real life. Detox regimens were in-place from the medical department. Psych meds were different.

After a moment to digest that comeback, he mumbled, "I'm not sure...I'm depressed about being here and need to get back on my meds."

"Well, you're in jail for manslaughter with a million dollar bond. If that was my situation, I'd be depressed too! Tell me what meds you were on and why."

"Well," head a little hang-doggish, "some anti-depressants a while back, then something to help me sleep".

"Exactly what was the last one you were on, when, and who prescribed it?" I asked.

He mumbled, "Hell, I don't really know, or remember; but I can't sleep in here, plus I'm really jittery."

With a touch of sarcasm in my tone I asked, "When you came in here did it say 'Albuquerque Sleep Center' over the door? You've done time before, so you know the drill, don't you? There's no such thing as solitude, privacy or sleep in here!"

"True," he acknowledged, as he began an attempt to convince me that he needed psychoactive medication for some mental disorder. Being a licensed mental health counselor, part of my job is to distinguish those with a history of an identified mental disorder from those who may be drug seeking, or fabricating symptoms to continue an addiction.

"This isn't your first time in a lockup, brother," I said, to let him know I wasn't a pushover.

He continued, "Truthfully, when I was locked up before I've always been on meds."

I countered, "When you got out, did you stay on them?" A positive answer to this is a good indication that one is serious about dealing with a diagnosed problem. Often institutions prescribe medications to keep a population sedated so fewer violent incidents occur.

"Really I...uh ...uh...didn't have the money or a doctor to write the script."

In reality, a correctional institution will ensure that upon release an inmate has a short-term supply of medication–enough to last until the person can consult a physician. But addicts would rather self-medicate than deal with the realities of life.

Our conversation continued, "So I'll bet you got your relief from the streets, didn't you?"

"Sure, it was easier and cheaper."

Looking for a deeper cut at the truth I said, "I'll bet that's how you've lived–the easier, softer way, right?"

His comeback was swift. "Sure, who doesn't?" He was sticking his chin out for a verbal right-cross.

"Your brothers and sisters in here live that way, too," I said. "Do you know that there are people who don't live that way? What if how you've been thinking and acting has gotten you in this situation?"

He was beginning to sincerely inquire, "What do you mean?"

I looked directly at him. "If you want an honest dialogue here, I'll only do it if you are no-bullshit-straight-up with me!"

"Man, what do you think I'm doing?"

"OK" I said, "Just checking. You let me know if I'm not being that way, too".

The dialogue went like this. "Do you think alcohol and drugs have anything to do with the mess of your life?" I asked.

"You're kidding? Hell, yes! From the time my parents split I started sneaking drinks. It was "get happy" time in Ohio. They were so pissed-off at each other that I fell through the cracks. By the time my mom found out what I was up to, I was shooting dope as a teenager. Then she tried to help, but it was like I was stuck in quicksand. She got me on meds while I was in treatment, but when I got out I was right back into it. I know it's an old story: my friends were all getting high, dope was everywhere and it was fun to just fuck-off. That got me a start on lockups. It wasn't fun, but not the end of the world. I hit the streets hard when I turned 18. It was just outside of Toledo in a little burg called Maumee."

"No! Did you go to high school there?"

"Yea, but I barely finished."

"I'm from there too. What street did you live on?"

"Shelly."

"Did you ever cut through yards to get to Holgate St. on your way home?"

"Sure. There was this one yard with this bitchy woman who would always yell at us."

"That was my mom, pal."

"No way! Sorry, man"

"No, It's true. She was. When she wasn't yelling at one of us she was yelling at some other kid. You took some of the heat off of me."

"That's amazing. I guess you owe me, then."

"Yeah, right. Tell me more about your history with real medications."

"I was on some kind of ADHD drug as a kid, which didn't work much because I was doing other stuff, too. Speed seemed to settle me down, but it was that heroin kick that got me. Somehow I made it through overdoses and all kind of shit. Now here I am. What am I doing telling you all of this shit?"

"Cause I asked, I guess? So, now what? Here you are, manslaughter charge, needing meds. You told me you're a junkie, I imagine you're detoxing. Welcome to the real world, man. You know, there's another way to live? Even in here, it can be different."

"Sure, people have been telling me that for 20 years. I never wanted any part of anybody's life. I'll bet you want me to tell you whether I did it or not. Most people want the juicy details."

"Really I don't give a shit! It's about you changing or not, that's all—and if there's something I can do for you..."

"Sure, get me some meds for this aching I got going on. I know I'm detoxing, but it's bad this time: chiva and speed. Not sure I'm going to make it."

"OK, Off to see the shrink you go."

"Wait a minute. Can we talk another time? There's not much decent conversation in here, none that's very honest, anyhow. Can you get me some paper to write on?"

"Sure, here's a couple of sheets; but what if I gave you a notebook? Would you use it as a journal? You know, keep track of your thoughts? I'd come back and then we'd have something to talk about."

"OK. But what should I write about? What I did? How I grew up? The shit I've done?"

"Write about your life to start with–you'll figure it out."

In a week or so I was back in his unit interviewing another person when he walked up to me asking if we could speak. Though I didn't have any extra time, this seemed important, and I said "Sure." Once in our private interviewing room he began.

"I got to the shrink, and what he gave me helped. Writing helps. Mostly it's about some history of using and crime. Is that OK?"

"Yep," I said. "Let's hear what you got."

"I've met a lot of guys in here, and our stories are a little different, but pretty much the same. Dope kicked my ass, and after a few rounds of probation I went to prison for an assault. After I got out a bunch of us were high and needed money for another score, so we tried to hustle a guy but he put up a fight and somebody hit him with a bat. Man, he went down, but didn't have much money anyhow. His brother was the DA, so we got hunted like dogs and I did five years. In there they put me on meds. Most of the others got sedated too, so we wouldn't cause trouble. It didn't matter 'cause there was dope in there as well. But that's when I first really paid attention to the recovery thing. They put me in an RTC (Residential Treatment Center) for a year, which was a lot better than general population. After parole I hit the road with this chick and was back on hard dope pretty quick. We ended up in Mexico, which was a little hairy."

"Did you do time there?" I asked.

"No, man. That's a bad place to get caught. We barely made it back to the states. My mom was in New Mexico, so I came here and tried to clean up, even got a job. But the dope life got me and I was living in an abandoned house–a shooting gallery. Almost died a couple of times from OD's. My mom helped me get to a detox, then took me in. I really tried hard to change, did some handyman work, was shooting heroin, then got in here."

"I've heard this story before," I said. "Tell me, do you think you're crazy?"

"Well, what's really crazy is how I kept going back to dope and crime. A part of me wanted to quit; but I just couldn't. I've seen guys do it, but I couldn't. No doubt I had chances, but I'm in here because of it."

"Do you hear voices or see things others don't?"

"I wish I did–it'd help me kick the junk I've been on. No, to answer your question honestly. I'm a junkie with a junkie mind."

"What does that mean?" I asked.

"Dude, I love the edge, and the street life–that's where the action is. The crazy part is the rush of it all, especially dope. You just don't give a shit after a while. "

"Someplace in you, you know that way of living doesn't work, right? I'll bet you've wished that it'd all be over and you didn't have to do this life anymore, didn't you? Do you know yet that something's gotta change?"

"Little late for that, isn't it?"

"You did the crime, now you have to do the time. But you have a say-so in how that goes; do you know that?

"What d' ya mean?"

"Over the years I've seen plenty of guys like you–well, maybe not exactly like you. You're brighter than most. You got time left in your life. Keep suffering, or not! There's a way out of your misery. I found it; and you can too.

Next I said,, "How about you write and let me know when you want to talk."

Given other emergencies, my concern for him slipped to the back burner until several weeks later, when I received a Request for Service addressed to me. Unusual. A quick check of the medical record showed that he was taking the prescription medication. That was a good sign. Though charged with a homicide, he was in a low security unit, and I could easily see him. I put him on the schedule to be seen immediately, wondering what was coming. When we next met in a private room on his unit he was a bit mellower, understandably.

Kenton opened our dialogue by saying, "I'm interested in what you said. How'd you know all that stuff? Nobody's ever talked to me like you did. What'd you mean, there's a way out? Do you have some secret way out of this place?"

"Yea, right. Like I'm gonna get your sick ass out of here." He snickered. I went on, "No, the worst part is that you are stuck in here with yourself, and 90 others like you in this Pod. You're trapped inside yourself. Hell, you were in jail before you got in here. Not only that, but you've been walled in, behind two feet of your own concrete. I'm surprised you heard what I had to say, let alone asked me back. So what do you want from me?"

"You don't beat around the bush, do you? I want to know more about what you said about that suffering thing, and what to do about it. My life's been a mess for a long time. Dope never fixed any of it. There's even shit in here that I've turned down. Now what?"

"Good for you. That's a start. Now, we'll have some talks, but you've got to do some work. I'll point the way. You walk it, or not."

"What kind of work? I've done that therapy shit before. It never took for me. Those people wanted me to spill my guts. I never trusted them."

"I don't care if you trust me or not or spill your guts or not. It's your life, pal." I pointed to my head and said, "I got some freedom up here, and not just because I get to leave here when I want. You want some peace? I'll show you how to get it."

"You don't care if I tell you my fucked up history or not?"

"Nope, none of my business. All you have to do is take some Good Orderly Direction. Or not. Let's hear what you wrote in that notebook I gave you."

After listening to his verbal vomit about how the world had wronged him, with no choice but the dope/crime life, I stopped him short. "OK. That's enough of poor, pitiful you. I'll give you some headings on these pages to give you a start."

I titled the top of a blank page, "What Got Me in Jail (not just this time, but all of the times.") Skipping three pages, I titled the next one "How I'd Like My Life To Be." I handed him the notebook and said, "That ought to keep you busy for a week or so. Oh, here's a book I brought you, *American Junkie*. Just read it, then write about your life. I'm not interested in how other people have messed up your life, but how you have; and how you've kept it going. Send me a note when you want to talk again."

A week later, as I expected, he got a note to me, but more surreptitiously than the last. One afternoon as I was headed north in the main corridor, a single file of orange uniforms was headed south. A fellow whom I didn't know got my attention as he approached, then pushed a small note furtively at me. Just like something passed between spies in a James Bond airport scene, I took it, not making a fuss. Being about the size of a matchbook, it looked like the backside of a magazine ad. Kenton didn't have to send it this way; like other inmates, he liked getting away with something. Besides, this was more direct, like "real-time."

Down the hall a hundred feet or so, as I passed through a rolling security door, my open left hand revealed the prize: "I'm ready. K." After a right about face, I marched across the main corridor, through another heavy security gate to "C" unit, right at the "T", into Pod #4. He was waiting. My ID got me into any unit, anytime–and out, thankfully. As usual, he was at a stainless steel round table seated with three other men playing cards, half serious, but mostly bullshitting. In the old days it would have been cigarettes for the ante and betting. Who knows what it is now, as tobacco is contraband. Seeing me, he nodded to an onlooker, who immediately took his place. Just another warm pair of hands. We checked with the C.O., who opened the locked interviewing room. Kenton took a seat. I stood for a moment, leaning against the wall while I did a quick analysis.

Kenton greeted me with, "Good to see you. Thanks for coming so quickly. I see you got the message by way of inmate postage. That cost me a soup. That's the price for getting stuff done in here. Writing is interesting and that book is an ass-kicker...my life, exactly. How'd you come by it?"

"My editor suggested I read it as an example of biography. After the first hundred pages it got boring, same old scams, dope adventures. There was no resolution, just war stories from the streets. I'm reading stuff more critically since I started writing seriously."

"You're a writer? I figured you for some kind of bozo shrink. What are you writing?"

"A manuscript about the Bubonic Plague which I survived in '06. I had to do it to make sense out of that experience for myself. It dogged me for years."

"Really? I thought that was all gone."

"Everybody says that. Now tell me what you learned from the book and writing."

"Man, for one thing, putting it down on paper made me less crazy–and I like doing it. Like you said, I had a part in all of the weirdness of my life. Here I've been blaming everybody else, especially my parents, for my shit."

"Right. Give me some details. It's my payoff for hauling my ass over here to see you."

"I think I was living pissed-off at the world, but mostly at my folks, and just found good times in dope with my friends, fucking off. Maybe I even wanted them to straighten me out, 'cept that life got a hold of me and it felt too good. Sometimes I wanted to quit and do right, but those straight kids were boring. Never really wanted to be a good boy, but not bad either. 'It' just got a hold of me, then it was too late once I found the needle. After that I did crimes to get money to get high. Probably I never learned how to be responsible and grow up, I guess."

"What about the part about how you'd like your life to be?"

"Well, some of it I'll never see, like a good job, house, old lady, nice ride. I'm probably going 'down' for life, so I can kiss that stuff goodbye."

"I'm not too interested in the outside-of-you stuff; more in the inside things. You know what I mean?"

"You mean like feelings and stuff, or something like accomplishment?"

"More like peace, less suffering."

"Sure, more of that, but also to not get so pissed-off, so easy; not bullshit or lie so much. In a way I'm tired of that, but it comes so fast. I don't know how not to."

"Sounds pretty honest to me. What other honest you got?"

"I know I've hurt people. My mom, my sister, and Katie, this chick who really liked me. I treated her like shit, got her hooked on dope, then I heard she OD'd. That made me real sad–I just got high to take away the pain."

"Did it work? Take away the pain, I mean?"

"Not really. When the dope wore off I was right back here in the same old bullshit life".

"You probably oughta do an inventory of all the people you've hurt, and those who hurt you, too. That keeps it from rattling around in your head. You're doing great, pal. Keep writing. Here's another couple of topics: 'How I Can Make My Life Better on The Inside by Doing Things Different on The Outside.' And 'Things I Can Do to be More Honest and Quit Bullshitting so Much.' See how that goes, OK?"

We parted with a smile and a hearty handshake. This went on for a dozen weeks or so. He kept getting more honest, expressing difficult emotions, sometimes shedding a tear or two. After his initial court hearing, he discovered a need for a deeper spiritual connection. As often happens in a lockup, inmates turn to the Bible for comfort and support–more like righteousness. He'd have none of that, so we investigated alternate forms of spirituality, which he embraced. Something happened. He started to change. As difficult as it was, he got more honest in his unit, even trying to help others.

Around Thanksgiving, I was dismissed from the job of two years. My employer, who had assumed the contract the previous June, took all of us employees on as theirs. In due time it was discovered that I did not have sufficient credentials to meet the requirements of the new contract. My layoff included a golden parachute plus unemployment compensation.

During my time off Kenton and I corresponded, enhancing our connection. While waiting for final sentencing, he was placed in an in-house rehabilitation unit, where he thrived, even becoming a mentor and remaining long after he'd officially completed the program. He finally got clean. The plea deal of a life sentence was pronounced in a hearing that I attended. That was difficult. He was not the same guy in front of that judge as he was when he went into jail.

By mail we've stayed in touch for a couple of years now, since he is in a New Mexico medium security prison. Since he'd had some training as a librarian in a previous prison, he got the job in the new one, where he can use a word processor. My life is better for knowing him: I have had a 50-yard-line seat, observing another person achieve maturity. Maybe there's a burgeoning writer in a cell in a prison with some peace.

Visiting Don

There's a first time for everything. Though I've worked in lockups on and off for 40 years, I've never intentionally visited a person who's been incarcerated. My circle of friends who might be in there changed 24 years ago. However, that doesn't mean my compassion for people behind bars is any less.

But to an employed professional, personal relationships with clients inside are anathema. Brightly colored smocks that said "Inmate" means "'keep your distance." Boundaries are boundaries, especially with convicts. There are too many stories floating around jail training rooms about staff being used to illicitly help those inside. Bringing in contraband is a felony, yet some personnel get coerced into it. Starting small with a ballpoint pen, the "game" can progress to taking out a letter, making a phone call, or sneaking in a lighter, tobacco, a telephone, porn or even a weapon. All have made their way inside at one time or another. I have seen it happen. Anytime they show up in a search of a cell, you can bet an employee ferried it in. This, most often, results in someone getting hurt if not killed... havoc for sure. The hoosegow is not a nice place. Residents are there for a reason, albeit sometimes unfair, as some claim. Caution has always been my guideline.

Nonetheless, there was a guy named Don in 'D' block in the Metropolitan Detention Center whom I got to know when I worked there. During an interview with him for a program in which I was employed, we had a direct, no-holds-barred conversation about his situation. When we first talked, all I heard was the unfairness of the charge for which he is jailed; and a lot about himself ("wonderful Don"). With a quiet voice I asked, "Have you ever thought that you might just possibly be a bit on the arrogant side?"

"Hell, yes," he immediately shot back, with a grin. "You gotta be to make it. But there's no call for what that bitch is doing to me!"

Once again he defaulted to his story about how the woman he had assaulted had responded. Legally, it was more like she got even. As the story unfolded, since this was his first offense, he was placed on probation. Per the conditions of his probation, the overseeing officer in charge of his case had inflicted restrictions on him. However, the "no out-of-the-state travel" limitation did not deter him, as a $50-an-hour construction job was calling from Colorado. Throwing caution to the wind, he went to Colorado, and a warrant for a violation of probation was issued. Nine months or so later he was stopped for a minor traffic offense. Friendly Officer Bob looked him up on the National Crime Information website, saw the warrant, and arrested him. The 500 mile long-arm-of--law in action, again. Several weeks later, via a circuitous route of small town jails and in shackles, he ended up in Albuquerque's Westside set of suites.

He is nobody's fool, and though not a big guy, he is nonetheless not one to be trifled with. When the courtroom dust had cleared, and his well-paid lawyer had been unable to ameliorate the results of the efforts of the judge and prosecutors, his yearlong adventure began. We met several months after he was sentenced. His well-managed rage sat in the interview room with us.

"All that may be true, but your ass is in here for a while, pal," my assertive voice came back at him. "Maybe you should use this time to look at yourself, especially your part in the deal."

To my surprise he seemed willing. "So what do you suggest?" came his question, not without a little attitude attached.

"You might want to look at your thinking. How your outlook and actions have contributed to this situation. I hate to say it, but you got your own damned self in here."

At first it looked as if my words might have ignited a short fuse. His quiet demeanor belied the mulling-over he was giving my words. Then, to my surprise he nodded and said, "You're right."

That was unexpected. I rarely get that response.

"Do you write OK?" I queried.

"Hell, yes. I've been to college." He said that in a tone that was elevated but mixed with some indignation.

"Then you know what a composition notebook is, I'm sure,' I said, returning tit-for-tat his almost snotty undertone. "I'll bring you one so you can put down on paper what's rattling around in that head."

"You do it, I'll do it," he replied curtly.

The deal was struck. He got up to leave the encounter. After taking a few steps, he stopped. Turning around he looked at me seriously. "Thanks", came at me in a manly tone, as he offered his right hand for a shake.

"You're welcome," I replied, as we grasped hands and shook tightly, man to man, eye to eye.

I knew I had a partner in the inquiry. Later that afternoon, I returned with a 100-page, 8 inch by 10 inch blank, mesh-bound writing tablet. That surprised him.

"You want me to come back in a few days so we can talk over what you've written?" I asked.

"Sure, I'd like that," he responded. Almost sheepishly he added, "I appreciate what you're doing."

Another firm handshake, then I left. Walking through the locked double-doors of his cellblock, I reflected. Part of my life's mission, this incarnation, is to help other suffering souls. Clearly, he is tormented by a past that is very present...like most of us.

The majority of us do not end up in jail; though we'd all be there if we had to go because of our thoughts. There is not a one of us who hasn't wanted to shoot, stab, or strangle someone, most likely a family member. For the most part we don't do it. Honorable values prevail, or fear of the consequences. In spite of feelings to the contrary, we do the right thing.

Life is strangely predictable that way: do good things, mostly get good things. Do icky things, one tends to get an icky life. Mess with the bull, and you get the horns. Then there are a few of us who can't easily tell the difference between the two (what's really right or wrong). It often takes a harsh comeuppance to point it out. Don was at that realization place; and didn't like it. Who does? Really, no one enjoys life inflicting a good 'ass-whoopin', then having to own up to the fact that we may have had something to do with the situation.

At some level, we all know that we are responsible for our lives. At least we have heard it one time or another, from somebody. How about this: Maybe we're liable not only for what we do, but what is done to us? Now that's a stretch. Few live that way. Don was on his way to this wake-up. YOU MEAN I MIGHT HAVE SOMETHING TO DO WITH MY LIFE?! He was getting a glimpse of this, like it or not.

A week later I entered his unit, unannounced. To my surprise, Don walked toward me as I reported to the Correctional Officer in charge of the 90 men housed there. (Now *that's* a job, managing these guys: no weapon, just a radio, phone and cameras.) He had his personal journal in his hand. With a noticeable nod to the left with his head, he motioned that we go to the attached recreation yard—more like an overgrown cage. Once outside we stood in the bright sun, leaned against the north wall, and closed our eyes for a moment, enjoying the natural warmth and light on our faces. Two guys sharing a special time. In jail even the staff doesn't get to see real light much, either.

"Well, anything show up in that writing?" I quizzed.

"Yea, it's pretty interesting. I can't help but be pissed-off at this whole thing. All I did was push her when she tried to grab my license out of my hand—well, maybe it was a little hard," he finally admitted.

I jumped in quickly," It's not about her—don't go down that tunnel. She's not here. You are. Don't get sidetracked by that bullshit. You gotta stay with your part. She may have tripped your switch, but you're no victim, brother."

"Whoa," he sputtered as his head jerked back. "That's a heavy word, man."

I bored in, "Did you get knocked around as a kid?"

"Sure, my old man used me as a punching bag till I got big enough to give it back to him. One good one and I put him right on his ass, then I left for good; never looking back over my shoulder.

You don't think this thing has anything to do with that, do you?" he asked.

"Maybe," I answered, in a questioning tone that didn't give away my certainty that it was absolutely true. Looking right at him through to the back of his brain, I said more softly, "It's something to think about. I've seen it in a lot of people."

"When I left that house I never looked back. Nobody was ever going to push me around, again. And they haven't until now."

We were in the middle of a pretty serious conversation; and he knew it. Thankfully I've been doing this long enough to know that saving someone doesn't work. Nor was he the kind of guy who wanted to be saved. What he got was understanding from a human being who would go toe-to-toe with him. He was enjoying this. So was I.

Then without hesitation I suggested, "Write about the abuse in your life, especially about how it's connected to being here, OK? By the way, I'd keep it out-of-sight. You don't want anyone reading it."

He seemed to disregard my caution:" No worries, man... anybody touches my shit, I kick their ass. They know it, too."

Trying not to be too taken aback, I stuttered, "O... O... OK."

He nodded, that thing which guys do with each other—sort of a wizened knowing between each other, meaning it's all understood. Then once again he offered me his right hand for a farewell shake. This time it was a less forceful. For years, as a carpenter, I swung a 32-ounce hammer, so my grip is pretty strong for a 66-year-old man. Experience has taught me how much pressure to exert and when. It's a manly thing; although I remember a female correctional officer damned near breaking my knuckles once.

"I really appreciate this–nobody's ever taken time to be straight with me like this. You're all right." He sounded sincere and humble. "It's about time that I deal with this, isn't it?"

In a similarly gentle way, I answered, "Yep. Thanks for letting me be part of this."

At this point we both knew this session was done. We sauntered across the terrazzo floor like two guys who owned the place...a sort of walk of kings. Savoring each step, having just been in the company of truth, there wasn't much to do but enjoy the present, which we did. A lift of the head, a glance at each other, then "See ya," completed that segment. It's moments like these for which I do this work. There's a place in all of us that is hungry for intimacy, even in the hardest "con." Knowing this, there is a practice that allows one to connect to that special spot. Not everyone lets themselves be so touched. Some ache for this union, being openly ready for the exchange. A good writer is hard pressed to describe a meeting say, at the grocery checkout when the cashier looks appreciatively, saying "Thank you." In that blink of an eye, before the "You're welcome," it can happen. There is little else in that breath than the realization of a link with another. Some might say there is a consciousness that a real person is over there, in those few seconds of time. I'm a guy who thrives on that kind of meal. Don was treating me to a front-row seat on his life. Now that's a real gift.

Between this conversation with him and the next, I was at my favorite little second-hand shop in a mountain community east of Albuquerque. As I perused the used paperback section, one popped out at me which I had previously read, *The Power of Now*. Though it didn't deal with abuse issues, I thought Don might benefit from it, because I had. His thirst for personal growth materials was growing. I'd previously brought him books, which he devoured, even sharing them with fellow seekers. Actually, he traded for coffee, since barter is the medium for goods "inside."

When next we met in our outside office a few days later, he was just as enthusiastic about our appointment. His toothy grin told me that he was still interested. Of course, when locked up, any visitor not in the orange-pumpkin suit is a welcome break in the boring routine. Jails do not typically provide time-killing activities, as do prisons. In state or federal facilities, almost everyone is kept busy with a job, mostly paying a dollar a day. "Dead-time" it's called in jail, just waiting for court appearance, or doing "short time," like Don---less than a year. He didn't have any relatives, close-by, who could visit, nor someone to put money on his account for commissary items that one would usually pick up at the corner store. Being indigent, as well as low-threat, he qualified for an out-of-pod work detail. Maintenance, like cleaning floors, or handling trash is performed by those living inside. They used to be called 'trustees', but that was changed when it became obvious that not all were trusty. He was a good worker who could keep his mouth shut, mind his own business, smile as needed, and do his time, though he'd never been incarcerated before. That surprised me. This was a guy who could get along OK, except in the area where his unfinished dramas of childhood caught up with him, like now.

When I entered his jam-packed pod a week or so later, he approached me as if he had known I was coming. He held his journal under his left arm and his right hand out for a greeting. There was a twinkle in his eye. Something was different. That's how real change is: clearly identifiable, if one is observant. Most people tend to believe another's words...not me. I trust patterns. That's what's really telling.

Then there's another essential ingredient: the observer's intuition. The term comes from the Latin *intuitus,* and means ""the act of knowing or sensing without the use of rational processes." Another way to describe it is "a knowing from inside." Think of it as a level of personal awareness developed through years of experience about damned near anything. Long-time workers in any field of endeavor have a special quality honed through repetition. Some call it practice. No doubt that's why there's the saying that "practice makes perfect." Successful people use it all of the time in their field of expertise. In my work, human behavior, I do for a living what others do for a hobby—understand people, especially anti-social types.

This guy, Don, was unlike others. Research abounds on criminals, in the field of study called criminology. So, why did this fellow, at 42, get arrested for a misdemeanor and sentenced to a year in jail, when others get arrested dozens of times, never doing a stretch of 365 days? Justice can be blind; but it saw him coming.

Somewhere, somehow in his developmental process he absorbed enough of the values of this culture to get him this far. The one(s) he missed got him jail time. His unwillingness to take a good look at himself has come at a price: jail, which he does not like. In truth, some offenders with multiple arrests don't mind being locked up. It's an inconvenience–the cost of doing anti-social business. Don minds; and when he got over blaming someone else for his situation, joined another whom he felt understood him, was shown a way to learn something that might help him in the future, he seemed to embrace a new path. Now he was ready for another lesson. It all comes in stages. He was about to get the next one by way of a collision of curious circumstances.

In between talk sessions I was looking at the Saturday morning newspaper, *The Albuquerque Journal*. I love doing the crossword puzzles, that's about all. But there, front page, lower section was a seven-column article about my guy Don. It was far from favorable. Written by an author obviously advocating for abused women, it included his picture–a mug shot–and featured a detailed story about the victim of his assault. Clearly the incident had opened a wound big enough for the New Mexico Legislature to climb into, bringing a new law to protect battered folk. It's no doubt needed. In New Mexico the spirit of the times is about protecting victims–not a bad context.

Don needed a lesson–not a bad thing either. Of all of the batterers on the loose, he's one of the less aggressive, this time. That mysterious Spirit of the Universe picked him for the lesson. His number came up. Bingo, you're in jail, now what? As he commented once, "God put us together in a room to see what would happen."

Back in the triangular shaped recreation yard with wire mesh for a roof, I asked him what he had discovered this week.

Like a kid who'd made his first work of art, he opened up. "I was in the wrong to do what I did to her; even though she might have deserved every bit of it. I guess it really could have been worse; but this is bad enough. Then I thought it was no big deal to take-off—arrogance, as you pointed out. I hate to say it, but if this hadn't happened now, with my hot temper, I might have done something worse later."

Pretty clearly he was feeling good about his self-appraisal. As I am wont to do, I saw a perfect opportunity to test his progress. Nothing like a monkey wrench thrown into the works to test the waters. All good teachers do this. It's been done to me. More than some kind of therapist, I see myself as a mentor of sorts. I decided to push the limits, not knowing the outcome.

"Last Saturday your picture was in the paper."

"Really?" He opened his eyes wider and tossed his head back a couple of inches. His response showed some surprise mixed with more than a little pleasure.

"Yeah, you've gotten your fifteen minutes of fame. The lady who wrote the article took what's-her-name's side. You seem to be the bad guy who got what he deserved."

In one movement he swung to the left, doubled his fist, hit the concrete block wall hard. "I'll kill the bitch!"

"Which one?" I countered quickly?

"Both of them," he shot back aggressively, teeth clenched, body tense.

I took a step backwards. "So much for your realizations, pal." I whipped back.

"Who do I talk to so I can get my side in the paper? Bring me a copy of that story!"

He reminded me of Yosemite Sam in a Bugs Bunny cartoon-snorting, consumed with rage, waving his hands, out of control. Or more like one of the Three Stooges spinning around on one foot in a circle, almost humorous. He was livid. "Slow down, brother," I said. "Look at you! Didn't take much to light you up, did it? You've made a really good start on changing; but clearly there's a lot of work left to do. So what's the connection to being so angry at women-or don't you discriminate?" Slowly the agitation subsided and the emotional storm abated.

"What do you mean?"

"Just because your old man knocked you around, why take it out on females?"

"Hell, I don't know. I've been pissed off most of my life." Next...silence. I let it be.

That's a really difficult thing to do, as most of us can't tolerate quiet in an interaction. Obviously, thoughts were percolating. Every human being experiences moments of profound reflection. Little does it matter where or when this happens: a promotion-a firing, a birth, a death, a special sunrise or sunset, or prognosis of imminent death. Or, on the positive side, having been saved from death, or a moment of deep intimacy. Something happens that causes us to pause and consider. For the most part, the precipitating event is unpredictable, yet tends to touch one to the core, momentarily. Often the shockwave lasts longer-like 365 days in jail. One is stopped dead in their tracks. Remember? I've had many; enough of them that I'm not so taken aback now. Every now and again, sitting motionless, asking for an insight, I'll get one. Instead of being hit over the head by one, I get a gentler nudge. Conscious relaxation lets them come easier. Research has shown this.

Neurologists liken this to the computer process of defragmenting a hard drive. In the case of human beings, it is the movement of memories (data) to spaces (neuron connection clusters in the brain) more appropriate for storage and simplification of access. "Post organizing," one of my professors called it. Integrating old thoughts with fresh ones to, perhaps, form an insight upon which a new and different future might be based. Most humans do not have much new possibility of what will happen next. The future is really our past waiting to happen again. Think about it. Well-entrenched patterns, often unrevealed, run our lives and are predictive of what we will do.

Don was now in a pregnant space.

"Holy shit!" he shouted, after what seemed to me to be much longer than it was. "My mom didn't protect me from him—I've been taking it out on women, ever since."

"Really," I responded as if surprised. "How's that?" Words practically fell out of his mouth.

"I've been attracted to women, romanced them until I got them; then they pissed me off and I went to the next—sometimes I had one on the back burner, waiting. My favorite song is 'Fifty Ways to Leave Your Lover.' You know, they've all reminded me of my mom in one way or another."

"Really?"

"Yeah, I was seeing another gal as I was trying to get rid of Rita, the one who got me in here. I think that got her when she found out. I can't believe how this is all tied together. Maybe I should thank her... but not right now. This is changing my life. I might have killed somebody if I hadn't gotten in here." Another long pause ensued. He continued, "Man, this is amazing. Who'd have thought...just talking and writing....."

We looked at each other for a moment, then I said, "There's another important ingredient: it's called willingness. Lots of guys in here stay pretty stuck. You opened yourself, didn't you?"

With a new element, humility, he responded, "True, but you are a big part of this. I wouldn't have gotten this far without you."

For once I was almost speechless. Then it came out, "Right! Now back to work. See you next week." But I didn't see him again.

The following Tuesday I was assaulted by a violent inmate who slipped out of his handcuffs in the middle of a group counseling session which I was leading. That guy got me good. Two weeks later, while I was recuperating, the phone call came from my boss, and his boss, that the program in which I was working was suddenly terminated. No more face-to-face access to Don. A few days later I got word to him through a colleague of my departure. All that was left for me to do was to write to him. After the explanation for the absence, I offered encouragement by mail. Within a week there was a return letter in my postal box:

"Man, am I glad you are OK I wondered what happened to you–nobody knew nothing. You disappeared without a trace... that wasn't like you at all. Then I got that note. It helped. At one point I wanted to know who hit you. Let me at him. I can get him hurt anywhere in here. I know people. Then I realized that wasn't right. Now I know you just gotta let go and maybe even forgive him, sometime; like I gotta forgive Rita. I'll tell you, I know how hard that is. Good luck on that, brother. Anyway, I'm sitting like you told me to. And I'll tell you something kind of weird. This is kind of hard to say, 'cause I never said it before, but I've felt it. I'm getting scared of getting out of here. Now I'm living right. What's gonna happen when I hit the real world? Then there's my son who I haven't talked to in 14 months. What if he doesn't want anything to do with me? I made some very stupid decisions that were all about me. Other people are starting to become important to me, now. So, I like getting your letters. When I got the one from you I was like a kid opening a present at Christmas. Thank you, friend. Don"

Now, I have to tell you: his letter was worth more than a year's worth of paydays. I'll keep writing.

No one can predict, for sure, what another will do, especially a guy coming out of jail, starting or trying to start a new and different life. Once a transformation occurs, life is wide open. But it's his deal, requiring vigilance, new values and a rigorous support system.

Oh, the visit. Trying to get in to see him didn't work. Since I'm technically still an employee, though laid off, I cannot go in to see an inmate. That's their rule in their jail.

I'm still waiting to be allowed into a jail as a visitor.

CONCLUSION? VIVA MUERTA!

The first few years after my discharge from the hospital, I made minimal efforts to address the experience. But it was always there. Every time I approached the touchy subject, emotion overwhelmed me. A year or two later I wrote a brief five-page story of what happened: the facts as I remembered them, and my reactions. Doing so brought me to tears. Four years after I got out of the hospital, my close friend commented that most of my conversation was prefaced with, "Since the plague..." I knew it was time to reconcile myself to it, and the way to do that was to write about it–not only my encounter with the disease, but the history of the plague across the centuries. The local library helped me with research, even obtaining out-of-state books. My hand-written story became the outline.

I've kept a personal journal and written in it almost daily since 1977, so I'm no stranger to putting words on paper. But crafting ideas into coherent sentences with an interesting twist for others to read–now *that* is the challenge.   My cheerleading squad badgered and cajoled me to trudge forward. Writing the first fifty pages was like pulling teeth, but my editor friend Barbara kept encouraging me. In February of 2011 I got the chance of a lifetime to spend six weeks in Lennox Head, Australia, on the beach in a beautiful house with friend Joe. There the manuscript took real form. Once back home, between work and the rest of life, making progress on writing about these events was challenging. I knew who to go to for clarity. Mr. Death had morphed into Viva Muerta, and I had a dialogue with him.

M: "Well, here I am again, miles and years down the road; and I thought I'd check in with you, Mr. No Bullshit."

VM: "You've changed my name I see. That's some progress. Perhaps I'm not the ogre you once made me out to be, eh? Nobody and nothing is simply black or white."

M: "Yep, I do get that. It's been an interesting ride since I first encountered you in that hospital room. As you know, I've written about that, as well as the trail of tales since. After all of these words about 'that,' I believe I've been trying to make sense of it all. What do you think?"

VM: "Before I answer that, tell me about this 'Viva Muerta' thing."

M: "OK, I'm 67 now, finally retired; and at this point, life looks a whole lot different. When I was a kid, life showed itself through very young eyes. At middle age, it sure was different. Now, maybe I'm not the victim of the flea–perhaps it was just some accident. But I've been an analyzer most of my life; like most of us, looking for meaning. Now the shift is toward getting the lesson from the experience. The truth is that everything comes and goes, including me. Life happens. So does passing on.

VM: "I take it you're looking at life with more maturity than blaming, as you did during our first discussion. Sounds like you took that little housekeeping lady's advice about getting to work at something; especially your own life."

M: "Yep. The bare truth is: (1) I was helping a friend; (2) I got very sick; (3) modern medicine saved my physical life; (4) friends helped pull me through with their support, and (5) I survived. The experience got my attention and made me recognize that I needed to make changes—changes that I didn't even know I needed. I felt the Presence of the Creative Force during the struggle to survive. When I was wheeled out of the rehab facility, I noticed the suffering on others' faces more. As I left, a fellow in a wheelchair was being taken in. Perhaps he once walked, now he didn't. I watched with different eyes. Everyone suffers, some more than others; however,

I've discovered a path out of suffering. I can't say that some blinding white light caused a 'rebirth,' but doing the next right thing, making adjustments by taking suggestions and being more open have made my life easier."

VM: "How philosophic. I got it all down here, son. What do you want from me? You're still on that side of the dirt, today. What's with you, always having to know? That's not where the satisfaction is."

M: "OK. Walking the line between acceptance and inquiry requires balance. Too much of either makes me nuts. Lately I've been wondering about passing out of here, and what's 'over there.' A month ago a guy, Brad, hung himself–he couldn't take it here any longer. His young daughters and widow have to live with that. Then last week a physician, Dr. Tim, said goodbye to this world, by his own hand. And he'd just gotten married a week earlier. That's a mystery. Imagine being that new spouse–maybe life insurance will take care of her financial needs, but cleaning up that psychic mess will take years and a lot of work. Those perpetrators of their own demise may have had some insight that the rest of us don't. Living with 'enough-is-too-much' just got to be too much. From my own experience of wanting out of here, I've discovered that the dark, ugly side of life can be intolerable; and at times I wanted no more of this world's shit. There's such a stigma attached to suicide. Conventional thinkers don't consider maybe, just maybe, souls chose to come here; then decided to go back. Or their time was up on their job here, whatever that was. Sure, it's conjecture. Esoteric writers, seers, and channelers say we're here for soul-growth. Maybe! It seems Pollyannaish to me. So, give me the answer, all-wise one."

VM: "Don't get snotty with me! It's everybody's choice. Consider, for once, that there's no right answer, just discovery. Or not. I've got no insight to this life. Pick a path that makes sense to you, then follow it. No, Mr. Pick-and-Choose, stay on the path! You want to get the real 'juice' out of life? Just be open, in this breath. You cannot change any of the past, at all. It was; and that's it. Willy Nelson was right when he sang, 'Nothing I can do about it, now.' Here's the real truth: Try really letting go, absolutely! Forgive everyone for everything, absolutely. Ask forgiveness from everyone to whom you have done harm. Try that on, daily, for a week."

M: "You're not kidding, are you? What happens after that? What's next?"

VM: "When all is said and done, when you let go of everything, I mean everything; there's only one thing left. And that's what you have been after."

M: "Yes?"

VM: "Just try it and see."

RUTHIE'S GONE

(A Journal Entry)
March 28, 1999

Last night Mom died. Ruth. Ruthie. But she always liked it when I called her "Ruthless." It gave her a kick to be joked with, except when the humor hit a little too close to the truth. Then she would retaliate with some kind of righteous attack. That's pretty human, I guess. If anything, she was full-tilt. Having raised seven healthy kids, she had sixteen grandchildren who loved her, and was married for forty-eight years to a man she buried in 1994. Her suffering ended yesterday when her body finally gave out. My buddy Mike says that she's a "Light-Speed Puppy" now.

Two months ago I traveled across country to see her, and found her looking pretty chipper. For the last eight years ill health plagued her. Starting with diabetes that was exacerbated by quintuple bi-pass surgery, she then lost her right leg at the knee due to poor circulation. However, she doggedly insisted that she could still drive. She never did, but was determined to do so; otherwise, everyone around her would suffer—and we did.

Often, she would get a pit-bull bite on an idea, throwing all of herself into it. Like when she took on her nursing home management. Since she lived in a Christian retirement center, she figured there ought to be a Catholic Mass there. She ended up eyeball-to-eyeball with the administrator, bugging him until a priest came in, biweekly. Then the whirlwind subsided, for a while. Mom always had to be championing some principle that involved a moral imbalance; and by God she was out to enroll anyone in her cause. Little did it matter who or what bothered her, she was not one to suffer in silence—nor fools gladly.

For most of my life her intensity alternately embarrassed or angered me—until I realized I am like her in so many ways. Only within the last few years have I truly accepted her. Finally being OK with my mom just the way she was took years to develop. Starting with toleration, I was able to work my way up to letting her be. I did not come into this world with much open-mindedness or willingness to see another viewpoint. She was that way, too.

Her critical comments left me feeling inadequate, and kept me from confiding my secret fears and concerns to her. I now see this was just her way of trying to help, and that was the best she could do. Her toughness came out in a tone of voice that was kind to others but harsh with her children. I feel more like I was trained, than raised. Despite the difficult process, the outcome was successful, as one of my sisters recently commented.

My years of tribulation with Ruthie suddenly shifted in 1996. When I left for a year's work in Saudi Arabia, before I boarded the plane in New York, I called her. We had the kind of conversation that I had always wanted to have: warm, sharing, supportive and loving. During that phone call I choked up several times over "thank you" and "good bye." She sensed my emotion, saying, "Ever since you were a kid, Michael, you have wanted to see the world. Now's your chance, son." All the while I was gone I wrote to her regularly, and called her every couple of weeks. When I went on a day trip, or met a new friend from another country, she questioned me for details– that was different. There was no inquisition; rather she seemed genuinely interested in and took pleasure in my adventures. When I think about it, she always encouraged my odysseys. It was almost as if she lived out some of her own unrealized fantasies through me.

My first real flight from home was when I moved to Montana in 1974. Dad and Mom visited my wife Jeanette and me in our little log cabin a year after we moved there. After raising seven kids, they finally got to have a road trip vacation together. And four years later when my marriage ended, they returned to Missoula to comfort me. That's when I first realized how much they loved me. We took some walks together, one of them on either side of me. Once we stopped on a little bridge crossing the Lewis and Clark River and we all embraced in tears. Even my dad, Mason, whom I'd seen cry once in all my years, shared my sorrow with wet eyes.

With her passing, I remember many other times that she showed her love and support. At the time, however, caught in my own wants and needs, I failed to see her generosity. When I was thirteen, I had an early-morning paper route. Though she often stayed up late doing laundry for nine people or cleaning up various messes, she usually awakened with me at 5:00 a.m. On mornings when snow or rain caused me to say, "Oh, No!" when I first looked out the window, she would haul my papers and me around the neighborhood in our beat-up old family station wagon.

Ruthie was a good mom. She certainly knew how to tend children. And yet she wasn't so adept when we got older. Control was the only tool in her child rearing kit. Yet, I now imagine that it must have been difficult to hold a screaming newborn while responding to teenagers' demands. "No" seemed to be her automatic-reaction to our requests. Still, at times she trusted this young boy. Occasionally I got to pedal my bicycle (purchased with the money I made from my paper route) fifteen miles across the county to swim with buddies at the Perrysburg pool, or the rock quarry where my cousin Tom worked as a life guard. Summers I got to work picking berries and to caddy at a private country club miles away, and she let me hitchhike way across town. I was only in the seventh grade at the time. Mostly I've taken for granted all of the love and freedom I was given as I grew up.

Now both of my parents are on the other side. When Dad died four and a half years ago, I was thrown into a crisis of faith inside of the question, "Where did my father go?" In typical Ferguson-sibling fashion, my sister joked on the phone, after she told me Mom had died, saying, "We're orphans now." Somehow Dad's death shocked me. Mom's death has had the subtle effect of leaving me lost and realizing there is an end to this life. I'm not concerned with where they are. I know their essence is with the Creator, in peace finally. They got their job done, as parents, showing me the way, and I'm glad.

A Week Later

The memorial service was held at St. Joseph's Church in Maumee, Ohio. Floods of memories mixed with emotions of loss and gratitude. The roots of my life were exhumed as we saluted her passing. Old aunts and uncles surfaced, along with cousins I hadn't seen for decades. Being with my siblings was God-sent. We cried and laughed like we did when we were kids. What I've missed over the years is our togetherness. We love each other. My brothers and sisters are profane, respectful, good parents to their kids, committed spouses, generous, law-abiding people who were trained to be that way by great parents.

What Mason and Ruth taught us I have come to believe is true: Life is all about The Spirit.

In New Mexico the flowers bloomed a week before she died.

Spring blossoms

Whisper the news:

Life goes on

ଔ

BIBLIOGRAPHY

Abbott, R., & Rocke, T. (2012) *Circular 1372: National Wildlife Health Center, Plague. Reston, VA: U.S. Department of the Interior, U.S. Geological Survey.*

Allen, A.,(2007). *Vaccine: The Controversial Story of Medicine's Greatest Lifesaver.* NY, NY: W.W. Norton.

Rosen, O. W. (2007). *Justinian's flea: Plague, empire and the birth of Europe.* NY, NY: Viking

Camus, A. (1948). *The plague.* NY, NY: Modern Library

Cantor, N. F. (2001). *In The Wake of the Plague.* NY, NY: The Free Press (Simon Schuster).

Chase, M. (2003). *The Black Death In Victorian San Francisco.* NY, NY: Random House.

Centers For Disease Control (2006) *Human Plague—Four States.* http:/cdc.gov/mmwr/preview/mmwrhtml/mm5534a4.htm

Centers For Disease Control. *Plague Publications—CDC Division of Vector Borne Infectious Diseases.* http://www.cdc.gov/ncidod/dvbid/pubs/plague-pubs.htm

DeFoe, D. (2001). *A Journal of the Plague* Year. Mineola, NY:Dover Publication. (originally published 1772).

DeSalle, R. (ED) (1999). *Epidemic: The World of Infectious Disease.* NY, NY: The New Press.

Drancourt, M. & Paoult, D.(Jan 2002). *Molecular Insights into the History of the Plague.*

Microbes and Infection, V 4, Issue 1, Jan 2002. http://www.macalester.edu/~cuffel/molecularplague.htm

The Black Death, 1348. (2001). Eye Witness to History. ,www. eyewitnesstohistory.com

Gregg, C. T., (1985). Plague: An Achient Disease in the 20TH Century. Alb., NM: Univ.of NM Press.

Helly, J. (2005). *The Great Morality: An Intimate History of the Black Death, theMost Devastating Plague of all Time.* NY, NY: Harper Collins

Johnson, S. (2006) *The Ghost Map: The Story of London's Most Terrifying Epidemic–and How It Changed Science, Cities and the Modern World.* NY, NY: Riverhead Books (Penguin Group).

Long, R E. (1994). *Ingmar Bergman: Film and Stage. The Seventh Seal: P.71-77.* NY, NY: Harry N. Abrams Publishers. A Times Mirror Company. New York.

Marriott, E. (2002) *Plague, a story of Science, Rivalry, and the Source that won't go away.* NY, NY: Metropolitan Books. Henry Holt and Company.

Moore, P. (2007). *Pandemic: The terrifying threat of the New Killer Plagues.* NY, NY: Citadel Press, Kensington Press Corp.

Moote, L. & Moote, D. (2004). *The Great Plague: The Story of London's Most Deadly Year.* Baltimore, MD: John Hopkins Univ. Press.

Orent, W. (2004). *Plague: The Mysterious Past and Terrifying Future of the World's Most Dangerous Disease.* NY, NY: Simon and Schuster.

Rosen, W. (2007). *Justinian's flea: Plague, empire and the birth of Europe.* NY, NY: Viking Slack, P.(2012). *Plague: A Very Short Introduction.* NY, NY. Oxford University Press.

"The Black Death, 1348"(2001) .Eyewitness To History, *www. eyewitnesstohistory.com(2001)*

Tysmans, J. B(1994). *Plague in India:---1994 Conditions, Containment, Goals.* School of Public Health. http:/wastetohealth.com/plague_in_india_1994.html

Zellicoff, A. & Bellomo M. (2005) *Microbe: Are We Ready For the Next Plague?* NY, NY: American Management Association.

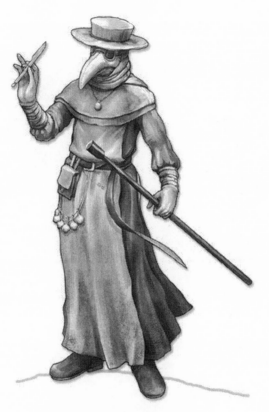

Community Plague Doctor

Plague doctors served as public servants during times of epidemics starting with the Black Death of Europe in the fourteenth century. Their principal task, besides taking care of plague victims, was to record in public records the deaths due to the plague.

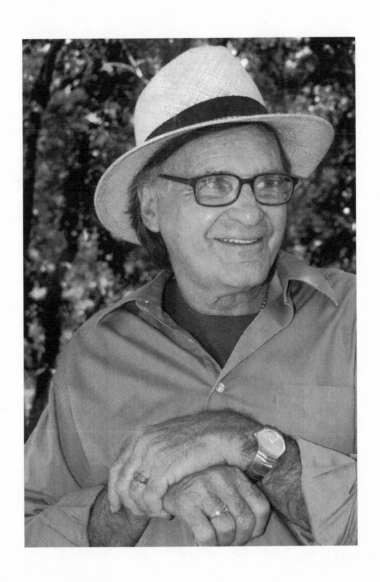

About the Author

In the throes of dealing with a life threatening disease, Bubonic Plague, Michael Ferguson received a blank journal from a concerned sister to help him in his recovery. In the process of writing, Ferguson found that he was recovering, or uncovering, the story of his life, a story of surviving and thriving that honors the millions who were swept away by the plague, and that serves as a model of courage and determined faith for all of us during these times of increasing uncertainty.

Michael Ferguson is not particularly remarkable in the circumstances of his early life. His parents, as he says, were good people—a somewhat emotionally withdrawn father, a histrionic and controlling mother—well meaning folks feeding children and getting them to school and church, meeting life in the '50s and '60s as best they could. Your basic co-dependent American family.

Just out of college Ferguson took a job in juvenile probations and, side by side with managing construction projects, has continued a woven path in the helping professions. Throughout his career he worked with tough and marginalized populations that put him in direct relationship with convicts and addicts, and that eventually led to opportunities in public speaking and training. There was only one small problem—he was caught up in the increasingly unsuccessful game of hiding his own chemical dependencies.

His successful and ongoing recovery with his own addictions that began in the late 1980s has provided Ferguson with experiences of deep surrender and the concomitant tools necessary for rebuilding lives. So in 2006 when he contracted Bubonic Plague, a disease that most people believe belongs to a dark age far removed from our modern society, Ferguson reached even deeper into that wellspring of spiritual waters. Some would site this second recovery as a "comeback," but in Plague No More the reader is shown a process of more than just surviving the mundane, rather a remarkable experience of being catapulted into a fourth dimension, a higher ground where life, all life, takes on new meaning.

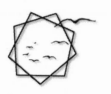

Made in the USA
Charleston, SC
28 February 2015